Soul Uncharred

CAPER BROWN

PAGE PUBLISHING, INC.
New York, NY

First originally published by Page Publishing, Inc. 2017

ISBN 978-1-68409-875-0 (Paperback)
ISBN 978-1-68409-876-7 (Digital)

Printed in the United States of America

This book is to all the people and organizations that have helped and supported me during this book's time frame. Organizations like Shriners, IFSA-(Illinois Fire Safety Alliance), CCI-(Canine Companions for Independence), Starlight foundation and Make-a-Wish, firefighters and first responders, and I'm not forgetting the nurses and doctors who performed miracles of healing. And to those who I've formed strong friendships with over the years as a burn survivor, you all know who you are, we may not be related by blood but you are all family. To my grandparents, to Bob and Dian Wells-my second set of parents away from home, to my foster family, and last but not least to family who has stayed by my side in spite of the difficulties that go along with doing so thank you everyone. Thank you to everyone who donated to my gofundme page, without your help I couldn't get my story published. And thanks to my brother Joey who might someday decide to share his experience as a burn survivor and perhaps more than anyone else-looks past the scars to see who I am inside.

Chapter 1

As I lay in bed one morning in the hospital sometime around late August or early September 1990, I don't recall if I was awaiting the dreaded morning routine or I had already finished it, but this particular morning, I noticed something I had not been able to see since four or five months previous. As I noticed there was a stainless-steel lamp next to my bed, I caught a glimpse of something, and I as looked closer, I could see eyes, lips, and very red swollen skin. From what I saw, I was able to discern that I was indeed staring at my own reflection. I remember feeling flooded by a whole series of emotions and thoughts about that moment as I realized I was looking at my own face. Was that really me? Oh my god, what have I done to myself? Will it heal? Will I get my real face back? I felt shock, sadness, fear, anger, disbelief, and a surge of emotion, which was just the beginning of a long road of healing that never really ended.

My full name is Capernicus Ray Brown, but everyone just calls me Caper, and I am the second oldest of six kids born from three fathers. Five years older than me is my brother Victor. Our parents are Ron and Sherri. Sadly my dad died in a truck crash a few months before I was born, so obviously, I never got to meet him. The only positive thing about not meeting him is that I was spared the pain of losing him. I can only imagine the pain Victor went through back then. Lord knows my mom still has her moments when she thinks about him, so I'm sure Victor does too. My dad's best friend is the father of Joel, but everyone calls and knows him as Joey. He is two years younger than I am. Then the youngest three are from yet another dad, Kirk Berg. First is Cassandra who is five years younger than me, followed by Elric seven years younger, and then finally Elizabeth. At twelve years younger than me, she is the only one born after *it* happened.

When I was about sixteen or seventeen years old, I had a disabled services caseworker who asked me, "Do you remember when you were little in the hospital?" Though I wanted to give a smartass reply, I gave an honest answer and replied with yes. The question offended me for a number of reasons. Firstly, I didn't consider ten years old as being "little." It might seem like such a simple innocent question, but to me it implied that I had always been a burn survivor and that it was the only life I'd known. I wasn't born this way, you know. I wasn't always stuck in this wheelchair. So when I'm asked a question like that, I feel that the person asking isn't looking past my scars to see the human being inside and the life I had before my burns. It was like negating my existence before my burns, so you might understand now why I find it offensive. I was like any other kid back then. I used to ride my bike, climb trees, and chase the girls during recess at school. Secondly, occasionally people tend to see me as being younger than I really am. It's kind of a double-edged sword. On one hand, my appearance doesn't seem to age, but on the other, people sometimes mistake me for being a child. Both subjects I plan to discuss further in my second book. And thirdly, last but not least, I'm lucky enough to have a very good memory going back to early childhood. I remember taking baths in a sink and living in a small apartment above a house full of girls. Heck, I even remember my crib missing two bars and climbing back out after being placed in it. I can even remember every house I've lived in, and we moved a lot. By the time I was burned at age ten, I had already lived in seventeen houses in ten towns and two states. The longest we stayed in one place was a little over a year. This is one of the very things that contributed to an unstable and already tough childhood.

If there is one thing I've learned about families, it's that every family has its own problems, be it the loss of a parent or both, drugs, alcohol, divorce, sexual or psychological abuse, poor income, poor education, unemployment, etc. But our family over the years had many problems. Most of those problems either directly or indirectly were a result of very low income. My mom didn't graduate from high school and, after she had kids, did not resume working. We scraped by with social security income from my deceased father and earnings from whenever Kirk was lucky enough to be employed. As for Joey's dad, he was never in the picture, so no help ever came from him. As a matter of fact, I had always assumed Kirk was Joey's dad, and I was twelve when I found out he actually wasn't.

When I was seven years old, I still lived in small-town Galva, Illinois, and whenever I was lucky enough to have some loose change, I would ride my bike alone to a downtown store such as Ben Franklin to buy candy. Or sometimes I would go to the park alone or perhaps meet a friend somewhere. I also rode my bike to and from school, usually alone or with Joey in tow. There was this one time when I was six, I came home from kindergarten at noon, and nobody was home. At that time, we lived in the northernmost house on the edge of town just across the road from the high school. But that day, I walked all the way back downtown by myself going into all the stores and innocently asking the clerks if they had seen my mom. It was as if I expected them to know me and my mom, but I was told no every time. I wasn't worried or scared as I went to the next store and asked the same question again. My last stop was True Value hardware store, where I asked again, and as the clerk stepped away, I grabbed a small Transformer from the window and simply walked out of the store. At the time, I didn't realize it was stealing and just headed back home. On the way home, I took the neighbors mail because I assumed it was ours, only for mom to tell me to put it back. Now if a kid did something like walking around town alone today, you can be pretty sure somebody might try to help that child because they assumed something was very wrong.

Times have changed so much since I was kid back in the '80s. All the things I did back then seemed like normal everyday life for a kid. I was very independent, and riding my bike to school or going anywhere alone didn't bother me a bit, and any danger was far from my mind. Partly, I think Galva was a great safe little town back in those days, but over time, society has just changed so much. Kids used to play outside all the time, either with friends or siblings, but now it seems most of them are glued to TV and digital devices. And then there's the fact that nowadays there seems to be more threats to kids, like gangs, drugs, bullies, pedophiles, and even domestic terrorism, whether it be a school shooting or otherwise. To put it simply, childhood isn't so innocent and safe as it used to be. Every now and then, I would come home, and Mom might be out for whatever reason, and it didn't bother me a bit. Left alone, we were just fine most of the time, but inevitably, boys and kids will get into trouble. This independence had its pros and cons. Obviously, the cons would be the bad judgments kids will make and the elements of unknown danger, such as a kitchen fire, accidental injury, or the many other accidents that can happen at home. The positive elements included teaching me to be independent, how to take care of myself, my younger siblings, and even the house.

Even though I was a scaredy-cat when I was young, I still would muster up the courage and go throughout the house on a stormy night, close all the windows by myself, and take the guinea pigs out of my brother's bed, or be protective of them and the house. Some of my most simple fears were of unknown sounds. When I was young, I used to be terrified of thunder and thunderstorms until I was about eight or so and town alert sirens even creeped me out. Now I'm an avid storm watcher and enjoy approaching storms, but the storm sirens on the other hand still freak me out; I honestly don't know why. Anyway, one night when

I was nine, I woke up to the sound of Cassandra screaming for Mom and yelling, "Freddy is climbing up my wall!" So I then yelled at Joey to take her downstairs to Mom. Meanwhile, I was still upstairs alone with my dog Rocky lying on my bed, wondering what was taking so long. I started to get nervous, and when I finally went downstairs to my mom's bedroom, I found Joey and Cassandra just sitting there alone. Mom, on the other hand, was nowhere to be found. At first, I was afraid of the possibilities of where she might be and what might have happened. This fear turned to anger when after some length of time she returned home from a midnight walk. This would fall into the con category, what if something had happened? I could deal with taking care of myself, but if something majorly bad happened, even my independence would not have been able to fix things. Some things like that would always require a responsible adult who could handle it. My mom did try to shield us from some things, but it was pretty pointless. For example, she tried to keep us away from anyone drinking too much around, but even at an early age, I was still a witness to drunken violence.

When I was five or six, we were visiting my aunt Judy in Knoxville. Later on, we had to leave, but I remember my mom said we were coming back. So for whatever reason, we went all the way home about twenty-five miles away in Galva then back again. By then, my aunt was overly intoxicated, and my mom decided to head back home, thus making a wasted trip. But not before Judy pleaded and argued with her to stay. I didn't care for the violence, but at that young age, even I knew it was stupid to go back and forth like we did that night. Don't get me wrong though. My mom, of course, will be reading this, and Joey agrees with me she did the best she could with what she had. Sure, we were poor and didn't have a lot of stuff, but we had her love, which is more than some families and children have.

Recently, I was going through old school notebooks from the months just before my burns, and I found a little essay I wrote about wanting to be a fisherman when I grow up, and it ended with mentioning, "I love my mom because she makes feel special."

During those first ten years of my life, I lacked a true positive male figure in my life. The only positive adult male in my life was my grandpa. For most of his life, he worked at the Burlington Northern rail yard in Galesburg, Illinois. From 1987 to 1990, Victor spent a bit of time coming and going, as he had his own problems to deal with. And Kirk seemed to be the same way but for different reasons. One day, when I was five, my mom was leaving to go visit him in jail. In blunt terms, I told her, "I don't like him, he's mean." He wasn't exactly the ideal father. He yelled, argued with my mom, insulted us, spanked, hit, etc. He never did what a truly involved and caring dad was expected to, for example, playing ball, fishing, teaching me about sports, encouragement, or basically just being a positive person in life. My earliest memory and example of him being a jerk was when I was about two maybe three years old. We were all walking along a country road with a creek on the side. He said in a mean tone, "Don't fall in because nobody is going after you." These kind of words stick to a kid, and I never forgot them. Or the many other memories like that.

During the summer of 1987, my younger siblings and I were placed in temporary foster care for a few months while my mom dealt with postnatal depression and issues with Kirk. Victor was still with my grandparents, but Joey, Cassandra, and I were all sent to the same foster home in Moline while Elric was placed elsewhere. They were actually fairly nice people when I think about it. Every Sunday and Wednesday, we attended church, and we also enjoyed a lot of camping. And when school started up, I earned a little money to buy cookies at lunch by doing chores like taking out the trash. In the meantime, my mom and Kirk moved from Galva, Illinois, to a farmhouse outside Annawan, Illinois. We finally went home shortly after my birthday in October, and until then, I never had to change schools, except for starting second grade at Moline. But starting with a class is easier than transferring to a new school later in the year, and Annawan was a big change from Galva. I may not have been popular at Galva Elementary, but at least I was still accepted. The new school was totally different, and I was often teased and made fun of for being poor. But of all the schools after Galva Elementary, it was Annawan that had been the worst because of teasing and bullying. Even some of the teachers there didn't like me. Once, I was threatened with a paddling from the principal after a girl approached me during recess and said I cut her with my toy rubber Indian tomahawk I brought to school. I didn't seek her out; she came to me and somehow cut herself on my toy. Go figure. She claimed she was cut, but I never actually saw any blood. And I was the one threatened with punishment. I never was the best student back then. And from what I remember, I didn't really excel at any one particular subject.

I had a few girlfriends through the course of those elementary years, but I never really was very popular. In fact, it was quite the opposite. Because I was poor and the fact that I was often a new student, I was a target to be teased and made fun of. But over time, I adapted and learned to deal with the teasing the best I could. Unlike some of the popular or smarter kids, I wasn't a troublemaker per se. I wasn't perfect. I admit sometimes I would get punished for horseplay or goofing off by not listening in class, but that was about it. Yet there were occasional teachers who viewed me as being a troublemaker just because I was poor and not a good student. Only once before I was burned did I ever get a detention. And that was for goofing off in the gym while the class was doing something. The class was racing mousetrap cars, but I couldn't participate because I didn't have one. And that was because my mom couldn't afford what was needed to help me build one. The last time I was in trouble before my burns involved an incident on the bus. I was jumping across the aisle from seat to seat, working my way further back. The driver warned me, but I still dared to go further back. I was caught, and as punishment, she made me sit in the front for the rest of the year. Luckily for me, we had a different driver in the mornings, and I sat in the back then. That just explains how I got in trouble for goofing off or not listening. But the popular kids would get in fights during and after school, receive detentions, talk back, etc., yet I was still viewed as being more of a troublemaker than they were. In my opinion, I consider this to be a type of profiling, and I still feel that it's one of the biggest problems within public schools today. For the most part, I never really liked school. I have a theory that could explain why I felt that way.

One day back in kindergarten, we were asked to bring in our favorite toy for show-and-tell. I was excited to bring in my Optimus Prime I had gotten for Christmas. I waited forever for Christmas to arrive and finally see it sitting under the tree, which by the way was one of the most memorable gifts my mom ever gave me as kid, so she did have her moments. Anyway, I brought it to class, and everything was fine until it was time to go home and I couldn't find my prized toy. I ran around, searching frantically as I started to cry with tears rolling down my face. All the while, my so-called friend Todd kept saying, "Over here, look over here, no look over there." Back and forth, I searched all over the classroom, but I went home empty-handed and devastated. Weeks later, I got what was left of Optimus back from Todd, who obviously had stolen it from me. I honestly think that left a scar on me and is a factor in why I never really enjoyed school after that. I didn't hate it, nor did I hate teachers or anyone. But that, combined with the teasing in later years, influenced who I was and would be in the future.

For a few years during the mid to late '80s, Kirk came and went. He was in prison for a few months during 1985, and in 1988, he moved with his brother to Denver, Colorado, to scout ahead for us to later move there. But there was one incident prior to Kirk leaving that just shows how their rocky relationship affected us kids. One night, Mom came into our room, telling us there was a fire. We scrambled, went downstairs, and got into the car. I don't remember when I fully realized there was no fire, but it was obvious when I asked about our dog Rocky and Mom said he was going to fight the fire. Then in the middle of the night, we drove twenty-five miles south to Galva, where Kirk was with a friend. I was too tired to remember any arguments they might have had, but I still paid the price of home instability the next day. When Mom dropped me off a few hours late at school, my teacher scolded me for being so late. It wasn't my fault I was late that day, yet the teacher assumed it to be. She never thought about what it might be like for me at home. One way or another, we were always eventually paying the price for instability that came and went.

On the other hand, one of my favorite memories from that summer '88 was the day Victor, Joey, and I went for a swim in the river about a quarter mile behind our house. It wasn't deep at all, and the widest spots were maybe only one hundred feet wide or so. That particular day, we decided to walk upriver a ways and explore as we went. I remember one particular part of the river where the mud was still freezing cold on the bottom. The cold sensation on my feet felt great in contrast to the record heat and drought that summer. As we continued our journey a good mile or so, we found a spot where huge carp were gathering in large numbers. The area was slightly enclosed, so while Joey and I tried to block their escape, Victor was catching those huge fish by hand. I honestly was too scared to do it myself because they were indeed so big. After he caught about six to eight fish, we had had been gone all day, and we had to walk back home over a mile through the dry cornfields in our bare feet. That part was torture. Had I known about it back then, I would have called it a death march. Each step hurt my feet, and the heavy scaly fish hurt my back as it seemed it took forever to get back home. Ironically, I didn't like fish back then, so I didn't eat any. Yet that is still one of my favorite memories of my brothers and me and a small glimpse at what our lives were like and our early independence.

We joined Kirk in Denver around late August or early September that year, and we then moved back before my birthday in October. I don't know why we came back, but we lived with my aunt Leslie in Farmington, Illinois, for just a few weeks until we found a house in Douglas, which was about twelve miles northwest. Kirk returned to Illinois sometime during the spring of '89 only to leave again a few months later after a fight with my mom and having an affair with the wife of his friend. The fight is one of those memories no kid should have to witness. I was at the table, eating breakfast one morning, as my mom and Kirk started arguing about something. They come into the kitchen, still yelling, and he pushed her very roughly into the corner of the kitchen counter. I could see the pain on her face as my mom said, "Kirk, not in front of the kids." And right there in front of us watching it all happen, he said, "F***k the little sh*ts." I never did forget that moment. Simultaneously I felt anger and helplessness. I was angry that he hurt my mom and the fact that he called us such ugly words, yet I was helpless to do anything about it. But once again he came back during the fall in '89, and by that time, Victor was living with a schoolmate in Henderson, Illinois. Even though the house in Douglas had a leaky roof, exposed rafters on the second floor, no carpeting on second floor, insufficient insulation, and crappy well water, for some reason, I still loved that house. To this day, I still have dreams of living there again both at age I was then and now. But in early 1990, we finally moved to Galesburg, Illinois, for the last few months of innocent childhood.

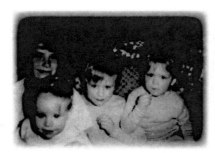 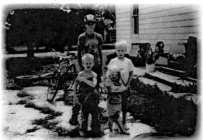

Chapter 2

Late March and early April of 1990 had their highs and lows. Sometime around late March, my mom had suddenly decided to give *my* bike to Joey. She told me Joey wasn't big enough to ride Grandma's bike she had recently given us. But I didn't care, and I was still very angry about it. I received that bike on my seventh birthday, and to this day, my mom still thinks Joey or Victor told me I was getting it for my birthday. That wasn't true at all. The entire summer of 1986, I wanted a new bike because my first one—a small Pac-Man bike—was run over by a neighbor's car. I was very excited when I received that bike, and I finally had something to ride to school and call my own. A bike isn't that much different than a car. It meant freedom and independence, with a bit of speed and fun added to the mix. I was always very sentimental and took care of my personal belongings, and that bike ranked among if not my top prized possession. So when it was given away with no regard for how I felt, I was nothing short of pissed off. I argued with her and ran to my room and lay crying on my bed. I then vented my anger and frustration on my bedroom wall. I kicked it a few times while my back was against it. Then I rolled over and saw two foot-sized holes in the thin cheap wood wall. Expecting a possible future punishment for what I had just unwittingly done, I cried a little more.

Around this time, for a few weeks, I was also pushing my luck with getting into trouble. When we moved in, I became friends with an older boy down the street who wasn't exactly a good influence. He, Joey, and I on the weekends would sometimes go downtown to the "arcade." Not the kind of arcade most people think of, though. This one was just a multistory older business/office building that at the time had an RC track on the top floor. We used it as an excuse for something to do when we (being me) were actually going to Walgreens to steal candy. I'm not proud of those choices, but on the other hand, I can at least say I never touched cigarettes, pot, or anything like that. And even to this day, I still haven't. Occasionally, I was also climbing the fence at the lumberyard down the street. I had no ill intentions though; it was simply to play with the guard dog inside. If I remember correctly, I think he was a large husky / St. Bernard mix maybe. Either way, I was trespassing, and yeah, that probably counts as getting into trouble. I was even testing the boundaries of risk and safety. That's kind of normal at all ages, but one day, I was almost hit by a car while riding my bike through an intersection without stopping. I was approaching at a fast speed, and as I entered the intersection, there was a screech of a car's brakes and a look of shock on both the driver's face and mine. I can honestly say I learned my lesson though and never did that again.

In April, like I did every year, spring fever was setting in, and I was already looking forward to warmer weather and summer break. I wanted to go the movies since the recent theatrical release of *Teenage Mutant Ninja Turtles* the movie and its solo hit song "Turtle Power." At school, I was also looking forward to a field trip to Wildlife Prairie Park before school was out. But before that came Easter break. Even though we weren't regular churchgoers, on April 15, Easter Sunday, our mom took us to church. And Kirk had to work that morning. Over the years, we would attend church irregularly, as if my mom was on a religious kick, gas costs, or whatever the reason may have been. We would attend for a few weeks or two or three and then just stop again.

After Sunday school that morning, I joined my mom in a balcony above the main sanctuary hall. It was taking forever, and I was getting both antsy and increasingly hungry. I asked mom if I could walk home to get something to eat. She said yes, so off I went. When I got home, I pondered whether or not I should make something for myself or do Mom a favor and make lunch. I honestly thought I was going to get in trouble for it, but I went ahead and made lunch. I boiled some hot dogs, heated up some green beans, and set the table—all without the modern miracle technology called a microwave. My mom got home with my siblings, and she was actually very happy I cooked for her. Her reason being she wanted enough time to feed us lunch before we headed out to Lake Storey Park for the annual Easter egg hunt. I was actually surprised by this and happy I could do something good for a little well-earned praise. I had always been very independent from a young age. It was just a product of my mom's parenting style.

There were quite a lot of kids lined up at the park when the Easter egg hunt was set to begin. I could run fast enough to beat the other kids, but I lacked a bag or basket for holding any eggs I found. As usual, I would make do with what I had. I used my shirt as a makeshift egg holder. Ready, set, and go, as tons of kids ran out to grab all the eggs they could, running and grabbing as fast as I could. Due to the ratio of kids to eggs, the pace of the hunt was actually very fast. And if you were too slow, you were out of luck. Toward the end, I rounded a big tree and spotted a final egg. I estimated I had about fifteen to twenty eggs already. But as I reached for the final egg, my stash completely fell out of my shirt, and I was swarmed by kids. Like vultures, they grabbed what they could and ran. I was left with three eggs. My focus, speed, and hope had all been futile as I threw them at the ground in defeat. As I was leaving, I saw the large pile of prizes and toys awaiting the kids who were lucky enough to have found an egg with a prize ticket inside. Why couldn't I ever win anything? I was always at the bottom, trying to scrape myself up off the floor and rejoice with some of the fancier things in life. My last Easter as a regular kid thus was a disappointment I'd rather forget.

We still had a few days off from school, and before our break, we were given a home assignment to earn a certificate at school for Earth Day. The teachers and school were in a care mood about the environment, and we were asked to pick up one hundred pieces of trash. I was half interested. I did and do still care very much about the environment. But as a kid on a school break, I just mostly wanted to enjoy my time off. I did do a little picking up around the neighborhood here and there. I even asked my friend Brandi to join Joey and me with filling our trash quotas. She then decided to speed up the process by filling her bag directly from the trash on her porch. Sneaky, yes. Did it work? Probably.

Victor had still been living with a friend in Henderson, but he was able to visit for a few days during Easter break. And I even got to see my cousin Nicholas and Aunt Lisa who had just moved back from Washington State, and that was the first time I had seen them in about three years. April 19, 1990, fell on a Thursday that year, and it was just another spring day. Kirk was at work that day, and Mom was at home with my sister and Elric. Sometime after lunch in the early afternoon hours, I was riding *my* bike around the neighborhood while I could. We lived right next to the railroad tracks, and on the other side was McCabe's scrapyard, which had two lots. One was on the west side of the street. This one had fencing, an office and building structure, a ton of junk, machines, and a crane in the main yard. The second lot to the east was mainly piles of scrap waiting to be recycled and processed. That day, I decided to venture into the west lot alone just for a simple curious peek at what it was like inside. I was very brazen getting in and laid my bike down on the ground just outside the fence in full public view and could even be easily seen from my house. Getting inside was easy enough because there was no lack of good-sized holes to get through the sheet metal fence. Once I was inside, most of what I could see were piles of scrap. There was a large magnetic scrap lifter crane, a very large sorting/shaking machine, random tools here and there, and a new red truck parked under a bay garage open to the main scrapyard area. I looked around for just a few minutes as I was checking things out. I even pressed the power button on the shaker machine. Immediately it turns on, shaking very loudly, which scared the crap out of me, and I feared drawing any unwanted attention, so I quickly turned it back off. Shortly after looking around a little more, I figured I had seen enough and crawled back out through the fence hole by which I entered. When I left, I decided I'd find Joey and tell him where I was and what I saw. After finding him and explaining a few details, he asked for me to take him in with me. I was already pushing my luck by going in once, so I told him, "No, I don't want to get in trouble." After an hour or so playing around the neighborhood, riding my bike, and the usual day-to-day stuff, I made that fateful change of decision. I changed my mind and decided to take him to the scrapyard.

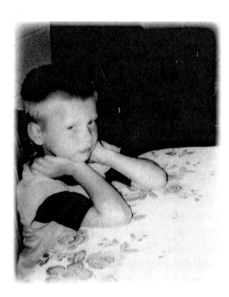
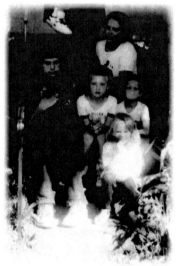

Chapter 3

We both laid our bikes on their sides so they weren't as easy to see and entered through the same hole in the fence I used earlier. Just inside the fence, there was an unused railroad supply line next to what I would describe as an elevated loading dock. The entire scrapyard is mostly level, but you had to climb the dock to get up into the yard area itself. I showed him around and mentioned the shaking machine. I dare not turn it on this time though. But this time, with Joey at my side, we checked out the garage and office area near the truck still parked in the garage. On one side was a windowed office with a locked door, and on the opposite side was a small break room. This door wasn't locked, and we went inside. As we entered, we saw it had a small table, sink, microwave, refrigerator, and bathroom. We looked in the fridge, and our eyes spotted a bunch of candy bars just sitting there. We ate some on the spot and stuffed our coats with the rest. Joey also noticed a few bucks sitting in the butter/dairy part of the fridge door. I actually told him to leave it alone. When you think about it, we were already committing crimes worthy of juvenile detention, so what are a few bucks more? But I still didn't want to steal the money. Ironically, I found out later on from Joey that he took it anyway. We left the break room and went back out into the main yard just in front of the garage. We noticed a gas-station-style gas pump just in front of the garage by a few feet. And we made yet another bad decision. Joey found a rusted hatchet, and we broke the lock off the pump. We then found some heavy work gloves, and I grabbed the pump as if it were a water gun. These details are still hard to talk about sometimes because of the guilt we have about what happened. For years, Joey and I kept these details to ourselves. I know I speak for him too when I say what we did back then made us feel like scum. Sometimes I think about what would have happened if we left before anything happened. Would Mom or Kirk have suspected or smelled something on us? What if something happened after we would have left? For example, an employee or two arriving and possibly being injured instead of us. I would not have been able to live with the knowledge that I possibly killed somebody. I was taught and believed that killing another human being is a sin punishable by hell. Anyway, I knew we deserved to be punished, jailed, taken away, you name it. I felt so ashamed, guilty, and stupid for what we did that day, but we both paid a heavy price with a reminder that will stick with us for the rest of our lives. I also need to point out that despite the rumors and the early stories and explanations about what happened that Joey and I gave, nobody influenced us in any way, and nobody ever told us what was inside. Nor did anyone come in with us at any time. Supposedly after it happened there were two other neighborhood boys whom we had hung out with sometimes and one of whom Joey liked to fight with at the bus stop who were rumored to have gone in with us told us about it. But our actions were our own; nobody else was involved. As I clearly stated above, Joey and I kept the truth private for many years before our guilt lessened enough for us to begin to explain the truth of what happened that day. After the pump lock was broken, I began to spray fuel all over the area. On the new truck, on the office windows, underneath the weight scale the truck was sitting on, even in a broken-down toilet sitting in a junk pile. If the pump hose could reach it, it was wet with fuel. I honestly don't remember the fuel having that gasoline smell, though. But I do remember it had a pinkish hue to it. I remember resetting the pump more than once, so who knows how many tens of gallons were sprayed. A safe guess in my estimate would be over a hundred gallons. I'm not gloating about the amount, just simply stating a fact. All the while this was happening, vapors were increasing and slowly approaching the pilot light of a heater in the break room. Suddenly, there was a quick flash instantly followed by a loud *boom.*

I was standing in the area just in front of the garage still holding the pump when it happened. Everywhere and everything in the immediate area I could see was covered in flames. I could not immediately stop, drop, and roll because I had to first get clear of the area on fire. I was completely engulfed in flames from head to toe as I ran far enough to get out of the fire. At this point, many things were happening simultaneously. As I was running and screaming at the same time, I was also thinking to myself I never thought something like this would happen to me. What would Mom and Kirk think? As I ran, I could also hear Joey's screams of terror as I began to feel my body stiffen up. It felt like my body was in a cast, yet I had never broken a bone before. So how could I know what a cast felt like? I reached the railroad dock, and I had to jump down to reach the ground below it. Finally, I found a place clear and far enough from the fire where I could begin to stop, drop, and roll. At this point, my memory begins to get fuzzy. Even though it's just one detail at this point which I don't remember, it was still an important one. Joey rushed to my side to help put the fire out. I don't remember this at all. It seems almost immediately somebody was able to get inside to help us. I lay almost naked on the hard stony ground, and I swear I remember this person or somebody else pouring water on me. Shortly after, the next thing I remember is my mom with me inside the fence. As we wait for rescuers to arrive, others are quickly making a bigger hole in the fence to get Joey and me out. I'm crying as I tell Mom, "I don't want to die." Those words echo clearly in my mind when I think of them. I know now how close I came to death, but back then it would be weeks and even months before I was fully aware of the severity of my burns.

Finally, I was placed on a stretcher and brought out through the now-enlarged hole in the fence. I was completely naked, and my scorched body was in full view for all the onlookers and gathered bystanders to see. As I was placed in the ambulance, all those people seeing me so vulnerable was the furthest thing from my mind. It was embarrassing yet at the same it wasn't, because my mind was in shock, and it went into survival mode, which sort of turned off that fear of embarrassment because it had bigger issues to deal with so to speak. If you've ever ridden an ambulance in an emergency situation, you might sympathize with this next part. After getting into the ambulance, I was bombarded by questions, many of which were asked more than once. "What's your name?" "How old are you?" "Is this your mom?" "What's your brother's name?" They asked my mom a few questions too. The first one was which hospital did she want to go to. I clearly heard my mom say, "Cottage Hospital." Coincidently, this is the very same hospital I was born in. The ride was fast, but the entire time, I was repeatedly asked the same questions. "What's your name?" "Do you know what year it is?" We arrived at cottage in less than five minutes and were rushed inside through the ER doors and into the emergency room. And that was when the real fuzziness started to set in. Because there was nothing for me to do but lay there as the emergency staff did their job, I could just relax and not worry about anything, so to speak. By this time, I was in very little to almost no pain at all. I've always been told this was from shock, but with burns of third and fourth degree, the nerve endings are essentially destroyed, and you feel no pain as a result. Finally, the last thing I remember is asking for a drink of water. A nurse told me I couldn't have a drink right now as I glanced over at Joey. We locked eyes as everything began to fade away.

Chapter 4

Galesburg isn't exactly a large city. It has two hospitals and a population of just over thirty-three thousand people. Neither hospital was equipped well enough to deal with such severe burns. According to my mom, I was only at Cottage Hospital for an hour until I was then life-flighted by helicopter to a hospital in Rock Island, Illinois, about fifty miles to the north. My mom tried to get up there as fast as she could to be with me. When she arrived, the medical staff told her my arms and legs had to be sliced open to relieve internal pressure and prevent tissue death by a standard severe burn procedure called a fasciotomy. After the procedure, I was then given morphine for the pain. According to my mom, the morphine was what caused me to go into my first cardiac arrest. I was then taken off the morphine drip and given something else to deal with the pain. I stayed at Rock Island overnight, and by the following evening, with the costs rising and yet still a lack of severe-burn specialized care, my mom and grandparents were seriously urged to consider sending us to a burn hospital such as Shriners. At this point, I recently learned that my uncle Brian was at the hospital and was trying to find out what he could do. Supposedly they told him I couldn't be sent to Shriners without the recommendation from a local shrine temple. With doctor's advice, Brian contacted the Mohammed Shriners temple in Peoria, and after being quickly approved, we were both then transferred by plane all the way down to Shriners institute for burned and crippled children in Galveston, Texas. Joey was sent first because he was stable, and they figured he would be fine flying there on a slower plane. They then flew me next because it took a little longer to find a jet to get me down there faster. So even though he left first, I probably arrived before Joey did. For years, Galveston has always been at the top forefront of pediatric burn care. There were other Shriners throughout the country, but Galveston was the first to specialize in pediatric burns. I was told many times during those early years by therapists and even my doctors that if I had been sent anywhere else, I probably would have died. This goes to show just how good they are at what they do. And all services and care from Shriners are provided free of charge. Expert care without the burden of debt saved my life. Needless to say, without organizations like Shriners, I wouldn't be here right now, the reason being my family would have collapsed from mounting debt placed on them by hospital bills and living day to day at my side. An already-low-income family struggling to pay hospital bills of massive unbelievable amounts would have simply been impossible.

My mom spent a lot of time praying in those early hours and days. Understandably, she went through many a night without any sleep while praying and worrying about me. She said she read to me while I was unconscious, and she carefully placed Q-tip swabs just close enough near my ear canals to absorb fluids that were draining out. She said doctors told her if she hadn't done it, I might have ended up completely deaf. Mom told me that the first time I woke up in Galveston, I said I was in no pain. I don't remember that detail, but my earliest memory after arriving in Galveston was waking up as nurses were rolling me to my side to change my bedding. I don't remember a whole lot of it, but I remember seeing the white of the bed, intense pain, and waiting for it to go away. That was also the first time I remember realizing, "Wow, I was badly hurt." But I still didn't realize the true extent of just how bad. Some people fall into or are put in an induced coma for weeks or sometimes even months. A few folks have told me there's no way I could have been awake in those earlier days, perhaps I was dreaming or whatever. But my grandma, mom, doctors, and others who were there know that even in those early days I was awake for short periods. I can't say exactly how much time has passed by the time I was fully conscious and awake. I know it wasn't long because of the details I've learned from my mom and grandma combined with the bits here and there that I actually do remember. But because of procedures and surgeries, any periods of being awake during those early days were somewhat intermittent, and so my memories and sense of time were staggered. Another difference between me and other burn survivors with serious burns is that I never had a tracheostomy. I've seen burn survivors with less visually apparent severe burns, and yet they were still "traked" at some point. In all my years at Shriners, I saw very few "traked" patients at all. I can't even recall any, which just goes to show how few there truly was. I always wondered why I never needed a tracheostomy, but my physical therapist Merilyn Moore said that was another miracle of mine.

I still remember some of the dreams I experienced during those early days before I regained a more steady consciousness. They were vivid, detailed, emotional, and lifelike. They all seemed to meld together, which seemed almost like no time passed at all between the explosion and when I woke up. Some seemed so real I could feel cold and heat. One of those dreams I remember sitting at my desk at school. But now the desk wasn't at school, it was for some strange reason at the Laundromat. I could hear sirens from fire trucks racing down the street as I put my hand around the girl at the desk next to me. I told her we would be okay, but we were both scared as I lay my head on my desk for protection from some unknown danger.

I also remember I had my feet propped up on a steel bar underneath my desk, and it felt like my shoes were melting against it. In another dream, I remember feeling a prolonged period of coldness. I was shivering as I lay somewhere, and I was repeatedly asking for a blanket and pleading for warmth but my pleas were never answered. In one of the weirder dreams, I was waiting at the bus stop for the school bus that day, and for some reason, I had my bike with me. I tried to board the bus carrying it with me, but the driver wouldn't let me on. And yet there was another dream I didn't know whether it was real or not, I actually asked my mom if it happened. Obviously, it never did, but I dreamed I finally got to see the *Turtles* movie at the theater. But as we were watching, I started to feel sick and tired, so we went home. These are the main dreams I remember from that time along with the bits and pieces too small to explain or comprehend. And they were totally different from dreams I experienced during surgeries in later years.

When the explosion occurred, I was wearing a gray faux-leather-type jacket. The best I can describe it was feeling kind of like plastic-like vinyl. I had heavy leather work gloves on my hands, jean pants, and black Jordache high tops. The jacket offered no protection from the flames and likely made my burns worse because it actually melted to my skin. Not to mention the candy bars I had in it that also melted. Much of those early days were spent keeping my burns clean, fighting infection, and recuperating from repeated surgeries. Infection can be a silent killer leading to organ failure and other problems. I was on so many meds and IVs that I later learned were likely responsible for my damaged hearing. During the first six months or so, I was constantly undergoing repeated medical procedures. This included excision of the necrotic skin / underlying tissue. And the accompanying skin grafts that would need to cover the exposed tissue. Only two places on my body were not burned. My hair was gone, but I was lucky that the burns were shallow enough that it could still be used as a skin donor site. These skin graft procedures were called autografts (thinly shaved skin from my scalp stretched out and placed on clean, viable, healthy tissue), from which the necrotic tissue had just been excised. My scalp would be used as the main donor site for many years. According to my physical therapist Merilyn Moore, who helped me fill in some of the details from these early days, "The healed skin from your scalp is ultimately what saved your life. The scalp area is very vascular [lots of blood vessels, so heals quickly], and it was used literally dozens of times [waiting for healing—ten to fourteen days between being recropped] as a donor site for the next skin grafting surgery." Ironically, the other unburned spot was on the soles of both feet. They were completely untouched, but the rest of it was so badly burned, I still ended up losing them.

It wasn't long after I was just transferred to Galveston when the skin grafting began and the life-changing surgeries were done on me. I had just woken up from yet another surgery. My mom was by my side, but this time, it seemed she had something to explain to me. She slowly tells me in no easy words, "Honey, your hands and feet are gone." What? No way! This couldn't be true! My arms are at my side with my hands folded across my chest where I couldn't see them, or so I thought. My mom continued to try to explain. I could see tears in her eyes, and I too started to cry. "Nooo, I can still feel them," and even to this day, I still feel every individual finger in both hands. Occasionally, I use them as a conversation tool, and I show others how I can even move them independently of each other as they see the nerves move in my arm. I cry and beg as I say, "They are still there a little bit." I swore I was still moving them as I grasped for the slightest hope that they were still there. I never knew the exact number of times, but according to my mom, I went into cardiac arrest twice altogether. I was asking her about some of those details, and she said it only happened twice and that the second time was during the amputation surgery. She also explained to me I had been awake in the days before the amputations were done. I do remember having an early conversation with her about where I was. I was sent to Galveston, Texas, because they were the best place to help me get better. I thought about the coincidence then, and I see it as kind of ironic now. In the days prior to the explosion, we were learning about the Alamo and other Texas places in our social studies book at school. Almost as if fate was warning or preparing me in a sort of weird way. The other thing I thought of was how similar Galveston sounded to Galva and Galvatron, who was a character in the Transformers cartoons during the late '80s. And speaking of fate, I used to be responsible for burning the trash when I was eight-ten years old. When I was eight I dropped a plastic gas container into the fire but quickly picked it up before anything could happen. And then ironically just a few weeks before the explosion I was burning trash again and a blast of heat burned off my eyebrows.

During the first few weeks after being burned, I received a care package of get-well cards from my entire fourth-grade class at Steele Elementary School in Galesburg, get-well wishes from people I've never met, and I think a few toys too. As the days passed, I remember conversations I had with my mom and grandma Barb about how Joey was healing because I was kept in an isolated private room apart from his. Because everything had to be kept as sterile as possible, all my visitors were required to wear a gown over their normal clothes and a disposable face mask. I remember those ugly yellow-tinted gowns clearly, even the SBI (Shriners Burns Institute) stamped logos on them. A little color and design on those things would have gone a long way. On one occasion, I remember my mom and grandma Barb entered the room and began to visit with me as they did something that upset the nurse. I think it had something to do with being on the wrong side of my bed because my neck needed to face the other way to prevent getting stiff in that direction. So the nurse ordered them to leave the room and come back in on the other side of my bed. They did so, but I always thought it had been a rude and rather weird request, especially of my grandma. I heard from my mom and grandma about some of the details of his daily trips to the tub room to clean his burns. Grandma still remembers Joey yelling in pain during his baths. She told me he yelled out, "Help me, Gramma! Help me, Victor!" or even yelled for my mom and me. After hearing those details, I did not look forward to experiencing it myself. During a visit, when he was allowed in my room, he told me they had a Nintendo in the playroom. I wanted so much to get better fast and heal enough just to go play, but that was months away from happening. Because of where Joey was during the initial explosion, he was luckier than I was. He received second- and third-degree burns to 28 percent of his body with permanent scars on his face and hands. I, on the other hand, fared much worse. I endured third-degree burns to 98 percent of my body. Mom told me doctors gave me a fifty-fifty chance of surviving, but it was probably less than that. So by all logic, I shouldn't even be here. More than once, I've found myself explaining the extent of my burns to somebody I've never met in person on an Internet chat, and they usually have doubts about my story. I am quite aware of how extreme it seems. I did live it after all.

Chapter 5

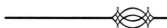

Until Joey went home, my mom and grandma Barb were my only regular visitors. Between the two of them, it was my mom who spent the most time with me while grandma was with Joey. None of my other siblings ever visited while I was at the hospital in Galveston. I did make an audiotape for them, so they would know I was "okay," but it was too far and cost too much for them to visit during my time in Galveston. From what I know, they were usually left at home with Kirk or stayed with my aunt Leslie in Farmington, Illinois. My grandma on my mom's side lived in Texas, and she visited a few times during the earlier days of my time there. My aunt Debbie on my dad's side from Tucson, Arizona, visited also. I asked her about my cousins Erin and Tony, and she told me they couldn't come. When Joey finally did go home after his initial stay of just over a month long, it was just my mom and me for a few weeks. All the while, I endured almost weekly surgeries and healing with no letup whatsoever. To make things more difficult, I was restricted to a fully flat position in a bed that could not recline or tilt. It was an air bed filled with sand, and when turned on, it was like floating on air. The restricted movement was necessary due to the grafting required for my amputations. Once again, Merilyn helped fill me in on the technical details of what was happening. "The second type of grafting that was used to cover your arms and legs [after the amputations] is called CEA [cultured epithelial autografts], skin grown in the lab from a few of your own nonburned skin cells. In order for the very delicate lab-grown skin to make attachments or adhere to your body, it had to be protected from shearing forces, from moving in bed, even with bandages over the top, and pressure from bandages, splints or just the weight of the limb on the bed over a period of time, which would prevent healing and possibly deepen the tissue damage. So your limbs [legs and arms] were suspended in skeletal traction [rods placed though the bone, and a harness with rope, pulley, and weights attached to hold the limb in the air], and your body was resting on the special air bed [called Clinitron]. Even with the best techniques and precautions, some of the CEA grafts were lost. Some areas had new CEA applied, and others were autografted instead using skin grafts directly taken from your scalp donor site."

I remember the setup and everything, but I didn't remember what its purpose was or if I was aware of the fact that it actually went into my bone. My mom even hung a few Ninja Turtle figures from it to provide something to look at. The bed was actually somewhat comfortable, but it was loud, and any body fluids or other liquids that somehow leaked or spilled onto the sheets resulted in annoying bubbling sounds, thus requiring nurses to change and replace the sheets with clean ones. But the hardest part of being restricted to lying flat was that I was unable to watch any TV. Without any visual entertainment, it made the days long, boring, and harder to keep track of time as it progressed at a snail's pace. I did at least have a small cassette stereo. I never had my own cassette player before, and the first cassette tape I received and listened to the most was Bon Jovi's *New Jersey* album from 1988. I've always been a huge fan of Bon Jovi. Proof of this is even in the only home video of my brothers and me, which shows me singing part of their classic song "You Give Love a Bad Name." Check out Fall-1988 on YouTube.

The other thing that made the months difficult was the fact that I could not eat. Due to all the medicines keeping me alive and my body unable to digest, any time I tried to eat even the smallest solid food, I would simply vomit it back up. But a body healing from injury or severe burns still requires more calories than I could get even if I was able to eat. So for a few months, I had a feeding tube in my nose. Every day I watched as the nurses filled the feeder, and more than once, I had the unpleasant experience of tasting it directly. It was nasty stuff, and the best I can describe it was being bad tasting, salty, room-temperature milk. Even their fresh cold milk tasted off to me, so the strange concocted drink was only worse. Quite often during the day, I fantasized of a drink. On some days, my thirst would get so bad as I fantasized about and craved water, milk, bits of ice, soda, Gatorade, or anything to quench my thirst and parched tongue. But for a few months, any drink would be few and far between. It wasn't until late august or early September about the same time I started sitting up that I was slowly eating solid food and enjoying fluids again.

Most of that first summer was very repetitive. Before I was sitting up, the amount of therapy I could tolerate was limited mostly because my grafts and body were still healing. While one part of my body was given time to allow grafting to heal, the other parts, such as my limbs and hips, went through painful range of motion exercises. The smallest stability I could count on was the daily morning ritual I had with my mom. Every morning when she came in, she would clean my ears, eyes, and nose with Q-tip swabs. It might not seem like much, but when you are absolutely unable to do anything for yourself, the smallest things really do matter. The itchiest part was dealing with my head after every surgery. Because so much of my body was burned, I had extremely limited places left on my body that could be used for skin grafting during surgeries. So as mentioned previously, for the first few years, the only viable donor site continued to be my scalp. After the skin was shaved, it was then covered with a Scarlet Red dressing. Scarlet Red is actually the ointment in it, but they referred to the gauze and ointment altogether as Scarlet Red. At first, it was somewhat sore to the touch, but it dried as the days passed and actually healed very quickly. As the healing began, it gradually itched like crazy, but it felt sooooo insanely good when it started coming off bit by bit, piece by piece, but never all at the same time. It was always bliss when it was coming off and one of the rare comforts I had in those days. The days dragged on with no TV and no food. It seemed I was having a surgery at least once a week to every two weeks. And to make things even worse, the hospital did not have AC either, so most of the time, I would have a fan running full blast 24/7 as I lay there mostly uncovered. Joey and my siblings were back at home with Grandma, and I heard stories of how he was scaring our sister with his new face mask. My grandma and grandpa took them to the circus, and life continued for them. But the days, which slowly passed by for me, were still dark and painful. I don't remember when the first one was given, but because I had been restricted for so long and did not eat solid foods, I ended up being given an enema for severe constipation. The first was unknown territory, but after that, I hated those things with a passion. I cried and dreaded them every single time. Since then, I've learned that what goes into them can vary. But I do know the enemas I received at Shriners were ultrapowerful and made me feel sicker than a dying dog every single time. I would throw up and basically feel terrible all without the privacy of being in a bathroom by myself. If I had been able-bodied, at least I could take care of myself. But no, I was in the care of others and completely vulnerable. A few years later, I found out that the doctors had actually wanted to do a colostomy. My mom knew I would hate this and refused it, thankfully. Obviously, such details are private and embarrassing, but I dealt with almost-constant bowel problems until I was fifteen, when I finally regained full control.

Even during those earliest days and months, there were a few staff at Shriners I was fast becoming friends with. I looked forward to these people because they kept my mind off other things. You could even call them angels in disguise because they do things that most people couldn't face every day as a career choice. Most of these "angels" were child life therapists and psychologists. Catherine Morgan was one of the child life therapists I enjoyed spending time with. She was awesome at her job, and I missed her when she left in '94. Bonnie Bishop was the head of child life. With Bonnie, I always enjoyed our long conversations about anything and everything. Even in those very early days, before I was even out of bed yet, she would visit with me for a chat and brighten those dark days. Patricia Blakeney is another name I must mention. She was a psychologist and had a very gentle touch and voice. She would stop by my room for a visit to see how I was, and almost every time before she left, she would ask if she could kiss my forehead. I remember her visits and long talks, but it's funny that only just recently, I remembered she did that almost every she visited my room, even during my later teen years she still did if I was laid up in my room and she stopped by. These individuals seemed to have a natural instinctive drive to care and listen to kids when they needed it the most. The earlier months, I was not yet dealing with physical therapists and the pain they could bring. There were a few nurses I was becoming fond of, but unfortunately, their job also requires the bringing of pain. Some brought a little more pain and discomfort, while others had more patience and better bedside manner. One in particular I'll never forget was Gene. He had a way of making me feel comfortable and just kind of hanging out, almost like an older brother or dad would, but in a cool way. Every time I saw him, I could expect him to say, "Downtown Caper Brown, what's happening, brother?" He was great, and when his job required him to do so, he almost always apologized for the pain. It may not seem like apologizing would matter much, but it did help at least. Less than a month after he went home, Joey returned to Galveston for his first clinical checkup. They checked on how his scars were healing and did some therapy with his hands. I heard from my mom he kept taking his hand garments off, but they were essential for reducing scarring and preventing decreased range of motion. My mom was looking forward to seeing and spending time with Joey. I actually was too, but it wouldn't turn out that way. As my mom and Joey spent time together for a few days I was left alone with no daily visitors. After three or four days of being alone, I lost it and just broke down crying. A nurse came into my room, and I then told her about my mom, and I was also thirsty. I was given a small sip of water to quench my thirst and luckily kept it down. When Mom finally returned, you can be sure I let her know I wasn't happy at all. This may sound a little spoiled and perhaps selfish, but how I saw it from my perspective, I was alone with no visitors, TV, or even food to bide my time. Yeah, I admit I was a little batty sometimes, but I dealt with it the best I could. More than once over the years ever since those early days, people have commented and asked me how I didn't go nuts from all the doctors, nurses, boredom, and pain that pulled me a thousand directions every day. I always gave an honest easy answer, "I don't know. I just did."

It was also during his visit back in Galveston that a reporter from KWQC Channel 6 NBC news did a report on Joey and me. Her name was Kate Worster, and my mom only agreed to let her in as long as I was kept off camera. She agreed and was allowed the exclusive to cover our story. I didn't see the report myself until almost two and a half years later. Most of it was focused on Joey's healing, his return checkup, and interviews with my mom, Grandma Barb, and Aunt Debbie. Back then, my grandpa was still employed with the railroad and, unfortunately, never got the chance to visit at the hospital in Galveston. Somebody always had to stay behind to take care of the family, jobs, and home. And between the two of them, Grandpa was the one who continued to work. While I was still restricted to a bed, the days seemed to drag on endlessly. I can't emphasize how much the most boring aspect of it was no TV. I would lay there as Mom described whatever she happened to be watching at that moment and wished I could too. For the most part, my only entertainment continued to be music. Bon Jovi dominated my small Sony stereo, but I also had Paula Abdul, New Kids on the Block, and the *Teenage Mutant Ninja Turtles* movie soundtrack.

I estimate it was sometime around July when I was no longer suspended by the skeletal traction rods. I think it was also around that time when I was being prepared and fitted for my first face mask. The purpose of a face mask is to control the scars from the burns and surgeries. My first face mask consisted of a custom-molded silicon mask placed directly over the face and held in place by a JOBST pressure garment on top of it. The mask only had small holes for the eyes, ears, nose, and mouth. Fitting it and putting it on had to be done very carefully because my ears and nose had been burned away and were at high risk for further damage if the pressure wasn't distributed equally to protect those vulnerable areas. Eventually, my entire body would require the JOBST garments, but not until my grafts had healed enough to handle it. It didn't actually hurt, but it seemed very restrictive and annoying. Imagine a ski mask you wear all day with about an hour or two break each day. It's as if it inhibited everything the face and head did. It got particularly uncomfortable and difficult if I cried. As a result, the mask made it difficult to breathe through or blow my nose after the crying. To make things worse, I was still on a nose feeding tube at that time too. And one of the scarier memories I have in that room before I was transferred to a four-patient room involved an incident with the nose tube. For some reason, I did not have a tube in my nose one day, and the nurses had to reinsert it while I was awake and conscious. As they started to guide it up my nose and into my stomach I started to cough and felt like I was choking, and I couldn't breathe. I began to quickly panic as I felt something wasn't right, and the nurses in the room reached for the emergency button every patient room had. I don't remember much about what happened after that except somehow nurses had handled things, and I was fine and calmed down. Luckily after that incident, I don't recall any other attempts at inserting a nose tube while I was awake. Though a few times I was threatened with it whenever nurses felt I wasn't eating enough when I had resumed eating weeks later.

Severe trauma can really affect your mind in a number of ways. After being moved to a new room, I somehow lost a few things I had been given. Including a stuffed bear my mom gave me I called Mr. Sugar. Before then, I had owned many stuffed animals, and I was actually sentimental about them, but Mr. Sugar was the first and only one I actually named, I don't really know why. For all I know, it might have already been on the tag. But when I was told it was lost after I was moved to my new room, I was crying like a toddler who had lost a favorite toy. I never acted so childish before my burns, so why then? Was it my own coping mechanism? As a way of dealing with all the trauma, loss of control, and pain, I had regressed to a younger state of mind. Though I'm an adult now, on the inside, I'm still just a kid at heart. I don't feel the need to accept societal norms and expectations on how an adult should act or behave. If it's not breaking a law, offending, or hurting anyone, even myself, then why should I? I still live up to and handle my responsibilities as an adult, but I still love to watch cartoons and be how I want to be. I've always felt part of the reason for that was, being burned had cut my childhood short. I missed out on things other kids grew up to enjoy and experience through the preteen and adolescent years. Watching cartoons, looking up old toys I used to have on eBay, listening to late '80s music are all ways I tried to reconnect with those final years and months before I was burned. I will explain more about this subject in my next book.

I don't remember if my mom had yet gone back home for the first time yet or not, but in the middle of the night, sometime around the mid-August or so, I was desperate for a small drink. The black nurse in our four-patient room that night told me I wasn't allowed anything to drink. I don't recall whether it was because she said I would vomit it back up or it was the doctor's orders because of a possibly scheduled surgery. Her answer didn't make it any easier for me. So frustrated with it, I started to cry and beg for even the slightest sip to quench my thirst. This in turn frustrated the nurse who then hit me on my right arm. I didn't know the rules about bedside manner, code of conduct, etc., but even though it didn't actually hurt, I knew she had hit me hard enough, and in a way, I knew it wasn't right. This just made me angry, still crying and still thirsty. She eventually gave in and gave me a small drink of milk. She was almost immediately correct in her previous assumption, and the result was me vomiting it back up. This angered the nurse even further, and she said, "See, you just vomited it right up." I didn't really care about how angry she was. I was just content with my thirst being temporarily satisfied. The exact date of when that incident happened I'm not totally sure of. I don't remember if I was still confined to a bed or if I was finally getting into a wheelchair yet. It was close to that time frame, but I do know that when I told my mom, she then told a head nurse whom I think his name was Paul. He was somewhat a tall guy and had a black moustache. He asked me to point out who hit me that night. I still don't remember her name and pointed her out in the hallways. She denied it, but I never did mention there was a second nurse in the room that night that saw what happened. I figured I wouldn't worry about it, and it wasn't really a problem. But for quite a few years later and more so in the first three to five years, there was a very small group of nurses who didn't seem to like me much at all. And one or two of them stood out from the rest. The others mostly seemed to change as I got older, for whatever reason that was. Perhaps I was easier to deal with because I was more mature and less needy than I had been in years past.

It was sometime after I was in my new room, albeit with three other patients, that my mom went back home for the first of three times during my initial stay at Galveston. The previously mentioned "hitting incident" might have happened while she was gone, but I know it happened while I was staying in the room I was in when she left. Neither of us remembers how long she was actually gone, but being alone made it seem like a month or more. But it was probably closer to half or even a quarter of that time. I was still fully restricted to bed, and I do know that she was there when I began to get into a wheelchair. I barely remember at the time though I was getting small opportunities to watch TV as I counted the days till my mom got back. There was no AC in the building, and I watched the weather channel and news with dread about how high upcoming forecast temperatures would be. The only thing keeping me cool was box fans operating full blast 24/7. I remember a nurse commenting one of the patients had a slightly low temperature because another patient and I had our fans going constantly. It was sometime around middle to late August when my mom was finally returning and my aunt Leslie and second-cousin Samantha were coming with her for the first visit since it all happened. All that day, I waited and waited as I began to worry something happened. *Is she coming today? Is she just late? Or did her plane crash?* It was late that evening when a nurse told me my mom had gotten in late and was at the hotel for the night. I wanted to see her, but I was at least grateful she was all right. What would one more night be until I saw her?

The next day, my mom was accompanied by Aunt Leslie and Samantha. Samantha's birthday was on the day after mine, so she was just under three years old at the time. This made her the first young family member to see me after being burned. I was still restricted to a bed and couldn't see her all that well. She could see me a little bit but was very quiet, and I'm sure she was shy and somewhat unsure of who I was and what had happened to me. The same situation would apply to my youngest brother Elric when he saw me. Samantha was younger than him but already talking about a full year before he was. Some of Elric's first words just in the few weeks before April 19 were words like *turtle power*. Over the years, I've learned I never really can predict how younger children might react upon seeing me. Some cover their eyes, while others might totally ignore my presence, and some might just simply stare. Or they may show their fear by hiding, crying, or clinging to a parent for protection. In the past, when it has happened with family or friends of family, most of them eventually outgrow, look back, and even laugh at it.

Chapter 6

This brings my story just about to the day when I finally saw myself that first time. Even though I wasn't in a room by myself anymore, I don't think I had seen any other patients prior to then. It was hard to believe I was looking at my own reflection. My face was deep red and puffy. My scalp was bald and was an even darker red from the Scarlet Red dressings. My earlobes were completely gone. My lips were oversized, and at the time, I was unable to close them normally. My nose was very open and seemed bigger. But on the other hand, I was lucky my vision was unaffected at all. Many burn survivors with severe facial burns end up with damaged eyesight or sometimes completely blind in one or both eyes. And some facial burns lack the symmetry my face still has despite still being severely burned. The thought crossed my mind that everyone must have kept mirrors away and not taken photos of me just to keep me from seeing myself, whatever the reasons might have been. I was no longer the ten-year-old I was just five to six months before. Before April 19, I faced the same day-to-day struggles any low-income kid might face. Teasing, bad influences, school, no money for candy or toys, etc., and now it was like being reborn with an entirely new set of problems and challenges with a new body to adapt to, just like an infant. I would have to relearn everything—how to feed myself, write, use prosthetics in place of hands, and countless other things most people take for granted. Not to mention the things I would no longer be able to do at all despite trying. There would be some things I just simply couldn't do for myself anymore and thus require somebody's help. I also thought I looked unhuman, gross, and hideous. How could anyone still see who I was inside and the boy I was before? There were photos of me at Starved Rock State Park from when I was eight years old taped above my bed. I often thought they were there to remind others and even me that I am still the kid they saw in those photos. I wasn't born this way. It's always hardest to explain to kids that I too used to be just like them in every way. I used to do all the things they do for fun. The younger a child is, the more difficult it is for them to grasp the idea that being burned from a fire is what made me this way.

My grafts were healing and were slowly beginning to tolerate more movement. Due to a vague sense of when particular events happened, I can roughly estimate when I began the slow process of sitting up and eventually getting into a wheelchair. It wasn't long after Mom returned from home after her first time being away when that process started. I was eager to begin getting up so I could do more than stare blankly at a ceiling all day with just my thoughts. I estimate it was late August when I was gradually getting used to sitting up in bed, then finally transferred to a wheelchair. One of my first memories of sitting up was watching a movie. I finally had some visual entertainment to occupy my mind and divert my attention away from how things were. Even though it was *Cinderella*, I was grateful to watch it, and cartoons would always be a way for me to concentrate on something other than pain or misery. Cartoons provided more than just visual entertainment. They helped keep boredom away, taught life lessons, gave me hope, and perhaps best of all, laughter. Rob Paulsen has been a voice actor since his first gig back in the early '80s. Some of his roles include famous characters such as the original Raphael, Yakko, Pinky, Carl Wheezer, G.I. Joe, Transformers, the Snorks, Donatello on the newest iteration of *Teenage Mutant Ninja Turtles*, and many others. He has a little quote I must share: "Laughter is the best medicine, and the cool part is you can't OD and the refills are free." This is so true for me. Without the joy, laughter, and hope I got from cartoons over the years, I would have gone insane. I've always loved cartoons, but you could probably say that it was part of my regressive coping mechanism, but hey, it worked for me. Getting up and out of bed also came with a price. My physical therapy was gradually intensified, and I was eventually fitted with the full-body JOBST pressure garments. The more I wore the garments, the more I noticed it changed the appearance of my skin. During those early days, I had areas on my body that resembled the diamond-scaled design of snake skin. But over time, this appearance faded away. The purpose of the garments was to decrease the inevitable scarring. With scarring comes skin contracting and tightening. That contracting is what made therapy so painful. I still had skin breakdowns almost constantly and quite often went back to Tubigrip bandages on certain areas to deal with blisters during those early months. Even to this day, there are certain areas on my body where pressure sores come and go for months at a time. It's just part of my life now.

Slowly as I was getting used to sitting up again, I gradually started eating. Just a little bit at first to get my stomach and digestive system going again. As I ate more every meal, I realized I was willing to eat almost anything, even some things I didn't care for or try before such as shrimp, peppers on my pizza, onions, etc. One thing is for sure, though. I used to crave for milk when I was dying of thirst, but I eventually did not like the hospital brand anymore. Simply because it just had a totally different taste than milk from back home. To provide my diet with extra nutrients, I was also given liquid nutritional supplements. These were administered in plastic syringes squirted directly into my mouth, and most of them tasted very nasty. Almost immediately after I began sitting up is when the dreaded morning bath rituals began. I had a few before I was getting up, but by this time, they were a daily routine. To be honest, I think this was worse than the therapy. I'm not afraid of water, and I wasn't before, but some people assume that my reluctance to get into a pool or body of water was because of my fear of water. That's not how it is at all. First of all, because of the severity of my burns, the water itself feels differently than on normal skin. Most of my body can feel the temperature of the water very well, especially my chest area. But even though I overheat easily, I don't get cold easily, unless the water I'm in is cold. I never lasted long in a pool because I got cold too fast. I never get into pools or spas anymore, and I'll explain more about that later. But the main reason bath time was so unpleasant was the pain. But it's not just any one part of the process. It was everything put together. Because I was basically helpless during baths, I was completely vulnerable and no control over anything. My baths proceeded like this: first I was laid on top of a flat bath table. It was basically a stainless steel table that was covered with a disposable plastic liner to drain the water. Most of the time, I was still bandaged as the tub room technicians then began hosing me down. They cut it all away and then came the painful wound cleaning and removal of dead skin. All the while, the tub room techs are talking up a storm with their Southern dialects. I have nothing against them at all, but me being from the north and in such an uneasy vulnerable position didn't help my discomfort. Those baths were the only few times I said out loud that I wished I had died. If that doesn't emphasize how painful bath time was, I don't know what will. The only comfortable part was after the bath; I was then transferred to a table underneath a heating lamp. It was amazing how relaxed that lamp made me feel after a torturous bath. Then I was wrapped back up with bandages and ointments and sent back to my room where therapy technician Ms.

Josey was often waiting to take me down to the therapy room for the next part of my day.

With continued healing and my skin becoming yet more tolerant, my therapy gradually increased in intensity. The intense therapy and healing was probably due partly to the fact that I was allowed a small window of time without any surgeries. Every day of the week, I spent five to six hours doing intense physical therapy. Early on, the main focus was getting fitted with the pressure garments, which would be followed by the first steps of my soon-to-come lower-extremity prosthetics. To prepare my legs for the new prosthetics, I began to wear lymphedema sleeves on my legs. These were attached to an air pump in an effort to reduce swelling and desensitize my skin. This would help me to increasingly tolerate more pressure. And then there was the prosthetics for my upper limbs. Other than me growing larger and needing bigger arms, the basic design really hasn't changed much since I started using them. I was fitted with two prosthetic arms with stainless-steel hooks that open and close when I move my arm forward. This movement pulls on a cable that goes around my back, thus pulling the hook open. The only thing keeping the hook closed is a simple rubber band. To this day, I use my hooks as a conversational tool for young kids. Many are afraid to put their finger in my hook because they think it'll hurt. I explain it only squeezes as tight as the rubber band, and I demonstrate on myself. And surely enough, there's almost always at least one kid willing to trust me and put their finger in the "line of fire." They soon realize it's no big deal at all. Ironically, even older kids and adults sometimes won't try it until they see a little kid who is braver than they are. Learning to use the arms was a very slow process. Because of my continued limited skin tolerance, for months how long I could wear them each day was also limited if at all. This made adapting and learning to use them slow. Therapy sometimes consisted of picking up individual wooden blocks and stacking them, playing with putty, and even drawing. Such things might be simple, but don't take for granted the things you do every day. Relearning to do even the simplest things was a daunting task. Learning to feed myself was as slow as learning to use them. But until I learned to feed myself again, I was reliant on other people during mealtimes. Food wasn't as enjoyable when I had to wait to be fed, and the actual feeding process itself was also tedious. The constant skin breakdowns on my body meant I wouldn't be wearing them all day until the following summer. And even then, I was still learning how to effectively use them.

Therapy remained an intense part of my daily schedule. But sometimes the relentless pressure and pain just got to be too much. Not only did I have to deal with the mask, but I also had to wear splints on different joints of my body to prevent stiffening and contracting. I had to deal with elbow splints, underarm splints, neck splints, and even small plugs to keep my ear canals open. I remember one day I was leaving the therapy room and headed back up to my room. But on that particular day, I was sent back to my room with a Thera-Band holding my arms closer to my body. A Thera-Band is basically a large stretchy rubber band used for physical therapy. It might not seem like a very big deal, but at the time, both of my arms were limited to a position where my elbows were straight out and my arms were extended out a bit from my side. Thus being held in this new position for an extended length of time was very uncomfortable. Picture the younger brother Randy from the cult classic *A Christmas Story*. In one scene, Randy is in his red snow suit and can't put his arms down. I was in the same situation except it was the Thera-Band holding my arms in place. As I got back to my room, I became angry and made my voice heard as I remember yelling about how Merilyn was to blame for my torture when in reality she was just doing what was in my best interest. Gradually, I would come to trust her as time went on and our friendship grew stronger. It was also around this time I began hearing talks and rumors that I was possibly being transferred back to an Illinois hospital so I could be closer to home and family. I heard Springfield or St. Louis might be where I was going and maybe soon. But these developments never happened, and thus, my hopes and short-lived joy were shattered, and I was again angry and frustrated. It was almost too much for any person to deal with. From early on, I had expectations of different things I would do when I got back home. For example, when I was still on bed restriction, I told my mom I couldn't wait to get back home for the summer so I could go swimming at Lake Storey. I know now she was avoiding the real answer, but at the time, she said I would have to be very careful in the sun and I couldn't be out long. I also remember talking about plans to visit Starved Rock State Park again and even the simple task of riding in the back of our station wagon when I finally went home from the hospital. All those normal everyday family events and things people take for granted, many of them I'd never be able to enjoy again. Finally, one day, my mom and I had a small talk about the reality and outlook of my situation. I faced many more surgeries and accompanying therapy. She also told me that I would most likely be in the hospital for a long time before going home and that it would be a few months until I saw my brothers and sister again. Hearing all of that hit me like a ton of bricks. I had fully expected to possibly go home soon, but then I had just learned it could be a year or two. How long was anybody's guess. I asked her about things such as when certain parts of my body would heal and when/if my hands and feet would grow back. At that age, there is so much a kid doesn't know. I didn't know what fire could do to the human body. Nor did I know amputated limbs do not grow back. After she told me all of this, I just remember I let it all out. I was frustrated, crying, and I told my mom, "The devil did this to me, and I hate him for it."

With the constant struggle and pain, which seemed to go on endlessly, there were things people did for me sometimes that helped brighten my day. Eventually, I learned these things gave me something to look forward to and kept my mind occupied and focused on the happier things in life. Within the first two to three weeks after being up in a wheelchair and not yet even fully dressed in clothes, I was told that there would be a surprise coming for me on a Friday afternoon. I wondered what it could possibly be. I even thought it might be something as simple and boring as finally being allowed to wear clothes on my entire body, thus being fully dressed. Nah, that wouldn't be much of a surprise because eventually that would happen anyway. When Friday came around, my mom took me to the playroom. I had already been going there almost daily since I started getting up in the wheelchair, but I was unable to actually play with any toys or video games at that point. When I entered the playroom, Bonnie Bishop was waiting, and the surprise was ready in the back of the playroom in the office. Finally, the door opened, and out came Raphael from the *Teenage Mutant Ninja Turtles* cartoon. He was my favorite of the four turtles back then simply because red was my favorite color and that was the color of his bandana. They took pictures, and he had a cart full of Ninja Turtle plushies to hand out to every patient. I was given one of each turtle to complete the set. The older you get, the more you wish you held on to certain things from your youth, and unfortunately, to my disappointment, my mom gave them away a few years later. But if I remember correctly, the picture of me with Raphael, Bonnie, and my mom was one of if not the very first pictures of me up in my wheelchair and getting back to my lust for life. Merilyn Moore said, "It was rewarding for all of us to see your vitality re-emerging." Over the years, there would be lots of little things like this which helped keep my focus off the sucky side of things by giving me something to look forward to or work toward for an enjoyable experience.

By mid-September I was just about back to eating normal food every day. A surgery was the only thing that disrupted my appetite.

For the first few years, any time I had surgery, I normally would not eat at all for two to three days or more. Back in those early years, every Wednesday evening was McDonald's night. Every patient was allowed to order whatever they wanted from McDonald's, and if they desired to, they could eat in the playroom. If it meant McDonald's *and* going to the playroom, you can be sure I accepted every opportunity to get away from my boring room. My mouth was still a bit tight back then, and so I was still unable to open it very wide. Not to mention I was obviously unable to feed myself at that point yet. This meant my meal consisted of Chicken McNuggets and french fries for easier feeding and eating. Even though it wasn't a cheeseburger, I was grateful to have it after the long months of no food at all. After the meal and helping everyone clean up, Catherine Morgan, who spent the most time with me in those early years, usually helped me build Legos, a puzzle, listen to music, or just talking and goofing around. Then it was back to my room when the playroom closed and any medicine or procedures that might be waiting for me that evening. The pain didn't end just because it was second or third shift and it was nighttime. There were still routines to be adhered to even in the early morning hours, anything from simple vitals being checked to dressings being changed two to three times a day. Nurses coming and going along with hearing kids crying sometimes and the room never dark enough for my taste meant the sleep quality could have been better.

Not long after the meeting with Raphael, my mom was headed back home for the second time. She had let me know a week or two in advance of her impending departure, but I was in utter denial and flat out said to her, "No, you're not." I actually believed by saying no and denying it would have some sort of effect and maybe she wouldn't leave. But the day arrived as I was still sitting in bed one morning while her taxi was outside the hospital, waiting to take her to Houston for her flight back home. The entire time, I was doing my best to get her to stay and denying she was leaving. In a petty attempt to guilt trip, I told her, "This is the second time you're going to miss my birthday." The first was my eighth birthday when I was in foster care. Alas, it didn't work, and the taxi couldn't be held up any longer. I was still crying when she left the room and walked left down the hall as I watched her through the window separating the room from the hallway. I remember yelling, No, come back!" and whatever else. Finally, I gave in and accepted it. I realized I had no say in it and told the child life therapist who was with me at the time to tell her I loved her. I don't remember who was with me in the room at the time because obviously I was distraught and emotional. But she told me she was sure my mom knew and loved me too.

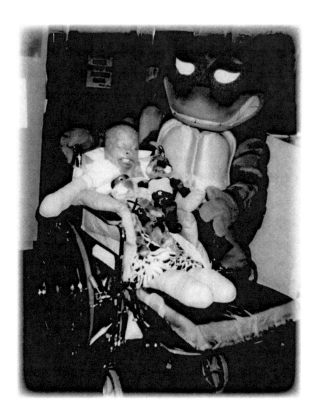

Chapter 7

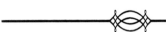

So now once again, I was alone in the hospital, but this time, I wasn't confined to a boring bed with no TV or food. And I had a room with three other patients. But a shared room had its pros and cons. There was help from other mothers and visitors if you needed it sometimes. For example, one thing I needed help with a lot during the first few years was being repositioned in my wheelchair. The early days were most painful because it didn't take much pressure to be completely uncomfortable. So quite often, I had to ask to be pulled up in my wheelchair so I could stay better positioned and comfortable. But inevitably, my position would change, and I'd ask for help, either from a nurse or (when I shared a room) from the mom of another patient. Other patient's family and visitors also were nice enough to chat with me sometimes. But on the other hand, I had to deal with limited privacy, sleep disturbances, and sharing a TV. The worst part in my opinion was probably the privacy. Not only did the other patients might hear or see what was going on, but so did patient family and visitors. More than once, I was in embarrassing situations where I could be seen and/or heard. It made me feel so small inside, which just added to my sense of vulnerability and loss of control.

While my mom was back home, Merilyn had talked with me about finally getting out of the hospital for a day outing. I looked forward to this and remember thinking I had seen and heard of vans with wheelchair lifts. That was before I knew manual wheelchairs could be folded and put into a trunk, while I was picked up and set into a seat. My first car ride and outing was with Merilyn and one of my doctors in his Porsche. We drove out to the seawall and all the way out to the eastern tip of the island. While out at this empty area, he gave it some power to demonstrate a small bit of what it could do. I was more excited and occupied by the car than by the sights and the town. Then we went on the ferry that took us across the bay to Port Bolivar. On the ride there and back, I could see Pelican Island and the remains of a shipwreck just off the edge of it. On another trip, I would get to visit Pelican, but after the ferry trip, we headed back to the hospital. All in all, I enjoyed myself and was glad to finally get outside the confines of the stuffy hospital and see what was beyond. Back at the hospital, as the days went on, my therapy intensified yet even further as my legs were being prepared for my first pair of lower prosthetics. Initially, the process started with me lying flat on a table and my prosthetics being put on. This first step was to increase my pressure tolerance and get my legs used to wearing them without any skin breakdowns or problems. Then when the time had come, the special table was tilted up at a ninety-degree angle until I was upright in a standing position. Whenever I think back to that day, I can't help but see the similarity to Anakin Skywalker's transition to Darth Vader in *Star Wars: Episode III—Revenge of the Sith*. Both of us survived severe burns and amputations of all four extremities. The table slowly rises, and from that point on, Anakin is no longer who he used to be. He was now Darth Vader, and the consequences of his choice and actions would be with him forever, just as it would be with me and my own. My life would never be the same, and in a sense, part of me was gone, and I was reborn again to start all over.

In the weeks leading up to and after my birthday, I was taken across the street to the UTMB (University Texas Medical Branch) campus to an audiologist. They confirmed my hearing had indeed been damaged and began the process of acquiring me a proper hearing aid. Shriners itself paid for it. It consisted of a personal unit similar in size to a cassette Walkman and a separate microphone unit to give to an individual person. The personal unit could be set to increase the volume of the sounds around me. This included all ambient sounds but wasn't good in loud places with lots of people and too much happening at once. This required the use of the microphone unit in settings such as school classrooms. It enabled me to hear everything the teacher said no matter where I sat in the classroom. But I still didn't like wearing it at home or when out and about outside the hospital. The hearing aids could be amusing at times though. During my early years at school, it used to pick up telephone messages in the area. And more than once, I had a teacher leave it on when they left the classroom to use the restroom. I even heard other people ask about the microphone they wore, and the teacher would explain it was for a hard-of-hearing student. But the most amusing thing I overheard happened many years later, which I will mention in the next book.

Finally, a day I was looking forward to for weeks had arrived. My eleventh birthday was on October 4, 1990. It was my first birthday since being burned and a world away from where I was just a year before. The previous year, my mom took my siblings and me to Walmart in Galesburg, and I was allowed two toys for my birthday. I had a thing for *Ghostbusters* back then, so I picked the Ecto-1 ambulance car and a figure to go with it. Then we stopped at La Gondola Spaghetti House for dinner. Those simple days were now gone. The night before my birthday, I couldn't have any food or snacks because I was going for an "unknown procedure" across the street in the morning. I woke up that morning, and the end of my bed had tons of balloons tied to it and my Raphael turtle movie poster was on the wall behind them. I went through my torturous morning bath and then was taken across the street for what awaited me. I think Paul was the name of the head nurse who took me that day. Before the procedure, we sat outside the hospital, which was just across the street from where the new Shriners building was being constructed. I could see the crane hoisting loads of mixed concrete to the upper floors of the still-skeletal-looking building. But then, it was time to go inside and see what was coming next. Of all my experiences over the years, that one was among if not the worst. I've asked a few close friends what the procedure might have been, but the closest description I can think of was a colonoscopy. I was on a table, and in a short fast description without too many private details, I was filled with a pink fluid that acted as a super powerful laxative, *and* a camera was then inserted. Oh my god, it was horrible, painful, and humiliating. No privacy at all while my bowel emptied itself on that special table with the specialists and Paul all watching and doing their jobs. I just wanted to crawl into a hole and hide. Thank God that procedure was only performed once. I had plenty of other unpleasant things I had to deal with on a regular basis without adding that one to the mix. What a start to my birthday. If that had to come every year, I would opt out of a birthday every time. That evening, there was a small birthday party for me in the playroom. We had cake, balloons, a few presents, including a copy of the newly released *Teenage Mutant Ninja Turtles* movie, and a large robot my mom mailed to the hospital for my special day. It had been a long day by the time I got back to my room. My mom called from home, and I told her about my day, waking up to balloons, the presents, and the finale was the movie I had waited for months to see. After the call, I immediately started watching the movie. I went to bed after the movie, and my first birthday as a burn survivor was over.

In the room I shared, there was a younger black boy who was burned less than I was. If I remember correctly, I think he was burned after getting into a bathtub of scalding hot water. Because his burns were less severe than mine, he was healing faster than I was. He had been in a wheelchair prior but was eventually walking and wearing his Ninja Turtle pajamas. He was even allowed to stay with his mom at an apartment while returning to the hospital every day for therapy and treatments. I noticed all of this and wondered to myself when I might be able to do all that. Within a few weeks after my birthday and before Thanksgiving, my mom returned to Galveston again. This time, Kirk was with her, and it was his first time seeing me since I began getting out of bed. But he didn't stay long because of the other kids waiting back home and left Mom here with me. Finally, sometime around November, I hit another milestone in my progress. Surgeries had slowed down enough to give me a break long enough that I was allowed to stay with my mom at her apartment just down the street from the hospital. It was a step toward returning to a life outside the hospital and apart from doctors, nurses, therapy, and medicine. I would sleep there every night and return to the hospital every morning for bath and wound treatment followed up by an afternoon of physical therapy. It was a welcome change of scenery from the stressful confines of the hospital. Just as good was the fact that it also meant I could finally enjoy more food from outside the hospital. During the day, on a few occasions, we went over to the food court at John Sealy (one of the UTMB hospitals) across the street from Shriners. The food court had lots to choose from, but the food was only half the fun. Afterward, we would go outside to the open court area and feed the pigeons and seagulls. In all my years, I never failed to attract a group of pigeons whenever I attempted to feed them. They would eat anything from bread, bits of hot dog, or even pizza. On afternoons and evenings, when my schedule wasn't occupied, we would go to the grocery directly across from Mom's apartment, stroll around the neighborhood, or even go down the beach sometimes. At the first souvenir shop we checked out at the beach, my mom bought me three souvenirs—a preserved baby shark in a glass jar, a white Gilligan's Isle–style tourist hat with Galveston on it, and a mobile of wooden hand-carved and painted parrots. My mom eventually donated the shark to a school, but she still has the wooden parrots. Every time I went to the beach, I wished so badly I could get out of that wheelchair to play in the waves. It was something I had never experienced, and I would eventually learn to accept that my burns meant I'd miss out on things I used to and never get to do some things I had yet to try.

Over the weeks, my mom and I stuck to a consistent schedule of bath times and therapy at the hospital while doing occasional sight-seeing and shopping during my free time. I can only remember one problem from our time together at the apartment. One night, I assume during my first few nights staying at the apartment, I just couldn't get comfortable enough to sleep. The bed was harder than my body could tolerate comfortably. It was just painful enough that Mom even became annoyed with me because I was keeping her awake. I cried a little bit, to which she told me, "If you don't shut up and go to sleep, I'm taking you back to the hospital." Her shouting didn't exactly help my pain or my feelings. After that night, I don't remember what was done to help me sleep better on that hard bed, but we had no further problems. Sometime around Thanksgiving, my mom and I went on our first shopping trip to Walmart. Our taxi ride was our first time in a car together after my burns and obviously my first time going to a big place such as Walmart. The temperatures were beginning to drop, and she bought a coat that I actually had a lot of trouble getting on. At the time, the best we could do was put it on me backward. I remember kids staring as my mom helped me try to put it on this way. Back then, it was weird having other kids look at me that way. But over the years, it would happen everywhere I go anytime I went out. I dealt with it as best I could by mostly ignoring it. Back then and even today, if anyone had the courage to ask a question most of the time, they would ask whoever was with me what had happened. I don't necessarily mind the questions, but it's the kids of any age who go to extremes to follow me and stare that bug me most. A stare here and there I can tolerate, but a kid who follows me throughout the store even if I try to stay out of view, lose them, or somehow make them aware the stares are unwelcome just anger me. The majority of those incidents involve a kid with no parental supervision who proceeds to literally follow me through the whole store. If I'm with somebody, for example, my brother, he is unafraid to verbally make himself known and tell them to go on. If I'm by myself, I always find myself wondering where the heck this kid's parents are. A simple stare as I am in view is tolerable, but following me throughout the store is just rude, and shame on them and the parents. After I got the coat, I also got a Bart Simpson shirt and a few *Ghostbusters* toys. One of them was a backpack gun-type toy that I wasn't even capable of wearing. It would take time to learn what kind of things I shouldn't buy because I would be unable to play with them. My eyes and my heart may want it, but it would often simply sit on a shelf to be stared at.

Not long after our Walmart shopping trip, Mom was yet again preparing to go back home, and it was also time for me to go back to stay in the hospital for another surgery. The evening I was admitted back to the hospital, I felt nervous. I enjoyed my time off from the stressful healing of surgeries. Now I was having another, and Mom was heading home afterward. That evening, my mom helped me into bed, and once again, the lack of privacy was a factor in why I still remember this. I was still having bowel problems, and without thinking of my privacy or dignity, she changed my diaper right there in full view of the slightly older patient next to me and a seven-year-old girl patient just across from me. Afterward, before my mom went down to the cafeteria, she told me to do some leg stretching exercises. On her way out, she told the little girl to watch me and make sure I did them. This pissed me off quite a bit. I didn't need a seven-year-old "babysitting" me and making sure I did as I was told. The very thought was degrading and offensive. I did them but took a small break after a few minutes. When my mom returned, of course she asked the little girl if I did them. She said, "He stopped." I glared at her as I explained I was resting. I really didn't care if Mom believed me or not. I don't blame the girl for it, but my mom should have thought more about respecting my dignity and privacy.

My mom left not long after my first surgery after those few weeks at the apartment. Once again, rumors and talks were spreading that I might be going back to Illinois. I very much wanted to go back but did not get my hopes up too much so I wouldn't end up disappointed again if it didn't happen. Therapy continued, and I also was finally able to play Nintendo. At the time, I was limited to playing Tetris because the game only required one hand. I was grateful for even this much because it was better than nothing at all. I was still actually unable to play with toys or stuff like that, and I gradually realized staring at them didn't really do much when all I wanted was to actually play with them. Then a few short weeks before Christmas, I received official word that I was finally being transferred back home to Methodist Medical Center in Peoria, Illinois. Part of the prior problems was that other hospitals and nursing homes did not think they could provide sufficient care for my needs. Finally, it was the staff of 4 Hamilton IPMR (Institute of Physical Medicine and Rehabilitation) at Methodist that accepted the challenge. In the weeks prior to leaving, my physical and child life therapists recorded videos of me to provide examples of my daily care, physical therapy, and leisure. The latter was to show them the boy inside, my personality, and the kinds of things I enjoyed. It mostly consisted of me lip-synching Christmas songs like *Grandma Got Ran Over by a Reindeer*, and before I knew of their fall from grace, yes, I even admittedly lip-synched a few Milli Vanilli songs.

My mom returned just two to three days before my trip back to Illinois. She brought Joey with her again, and that was the first time we got to see and spend time together since I was no longer bedridden. It was great to see him after being without my siblings for so long. But I heard he was still struggling with keeping his face mask and glove garments on. He had the ability to remove them if he wanted to; I didn't. I think it was a Saturday, and the same day, they returned that the Shriners had a Christmas party in the small atrium room at the hospital. Santa was obviously there with elves and the Shriners with their traditional red fez hats. They were distributing toys to all the patients at the hospital. Once again, this was an example of the dedication of the Shriners to the children to keep their spirits up. Happiness and laughter is the best medicine. I was given a plush Garfield and some

Micro Machines, which Joey ended up taking home with him because I was leaving soon anyway. In all my years and months I stayed at Galveston over the years, I never did spend a Christmas down there. Though there were a few Thanksgivings. The following day, my therapist Merilyn, my mom, Joey, and I went on a day trip to Seawolf Park on Pelican Island. The park is a memorial to the USS *Seawolf* and has a submarine and destroyer for public tours. Ironically, just before I was burned, I checked out a book all about submarines from my school library. I actually still had it when the explosion happened. There was a ramp for getting atop the submarine and tourist binoculars on a stand positioned on the bow of the sub. My mom and Joey went down and inside the sub to look around. I was eager to go inside and had an idea of the layout of the sub, and I wanted to see the torpedo room, but this would be my first time seeing my brother do something while I was left behind. A wheelchair obviously had no equal access to the inside of a navy submarine, nor the destroyer nearby. It was difficult being left out, but those restrictions were just another difficult aspect of my new life I would eventually learn to accept. But at least I was able to use the binoculars to watch a wild dolphin racing a huge oil tanker. I had never seen a dolphin before, either wild or captive. Seeing it in action at least helped lessen my frustration of not being able to go inside the sub.

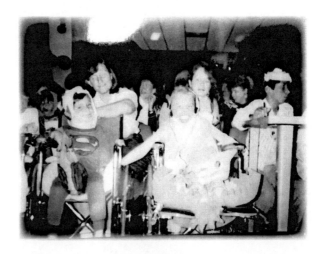

Chapter 8

On December 12, 1990, the long-awaited day had finally arrived. Even better, I was excited to go back home to Illinois before Christmas arrived. Not only that, but it would also be my first time flying while awake. So in essence, it was like I was flying for my first time. I would also be closer to my family so they could visit more, and I'd be able to enjoy the snow of winter. At the same time, I must admit there was a small amount of anxiety about going to a new hospital. A new hospital meant new faces, relearning routines, and different ways of doing things. My mom and Joey were flying back the day after me, so Merilyn accompanied me on my flight. She was also coming along to teach the new staff about my different needs, such as therapy, baths, wound care, etc. Merilyn even made sure my first flight went smoothly and brought chewing gum and a small handheld game. But I was actually more occupied by the airplane and the flight itself. We left Galveston at about five that morning so that we would arrive on time at Hobby Airport in Houston. I still remember the first take off, and as we climbed into the air, I felt the thump of the landing gear as it folded into the plane. Then not long after that, the plane suddenly jerked up and down. My eyes went wide, and I wondered just what the heck was going on. I didn't survive an explosion just to end up being killed in a plane crash. I learned it was turbulence and just a normal part of flying. Our flight took us to St. Louis for our first stop before continuing to Peoria. As we disembarked the plane, the pilot and crew gave me the flight plan map as a souvenir of my first flight, and then we headed off to find our plane to Peoria. The second leg of our trip was a lot shorter than the first, and before we had time to relax and enjoy a can of ginger ale, we were already descending for the landing. Finally, I arrived back in Illinois, and when I got off the plane, boy did I feel it. Immediately, the air was crisp and much colder, and that's how I knew I was home. We were greeted inside by some Shriners from the local Mohammed Temple and Methodist staff. For the most part, our flight went off without a hitch, but we discovered that we had arrived without half of our luggage, including the bag carrying my prosthetic legs. I don't actually remember that, but Merilyn told me I cheered when I was told my legs were missing.

On the car ride to Methodist, I remember the feelings of apprehension and nervousness about the unknown elements of the new transition. All the while, I stared out the windows of the car and took notice of the area because prior to then, I had only been to Peoria about three to four times in my entire life. But once I've been somewhere I quickly know my way around, and for my age, I had a better sense of direction than most adults, and that's not an exaggeration. So I tend to get annoyed whenever somebody is afraid of getting lost or ignores my directional advice. After we arrived at Methodist, we were greeted and escorted up to the rehab floor as it was then known as 4 Hamilton. Upon my arrival, I could see Christmas decorations, nurses, therapists, and older patients everywhere. For the most part, I was on a floor full of "old people." Most of them were seniors who had suffered strokes or injuries requiring rehabilitation, such as hip injuries from a fall. But there was also a small few who sustained paralyzing injuries in accidents. When I was admitted, my first room was shared with a guy named Billy, who was paralyzed from the waist down in a football game. I may have started out nervous, but I would soon learn that all of the patients and staff at Methodist were great to me and I couldn't have picked a better hospital to be transferred to. I do look back sometimes and think my age might have had something to do with that. Of course, my situation meant I faced many challenges, and my strength inspired others, but I also think because I was indeed the youngest on the floor, it gave the staff a change of pace apart from working with seniors and simply brought a little more fun and positive "light" into their lives.

Almost immediately after I arrived at Methodist, within a few weeks or so, I was given a power wheelchair. The process of acquiring one for me had actually begun before I even left Shriners. I loved regaining some of my independence. I no longer had to rely on anyone to get around or sit around in the same boring spot for hour after hour. And when I was moving, I was flying. I had a need for speed. Why go slow when I could fly down the halls with the same effort? I never did hit anyone, and I quickly earned the nickname Hot Rod. A nurse's aide named Diane Wells gave me the nickname. From very early on, Diane and I seemed to become attached. And as we grew closer, I eventually considered her to be my second mother. It made sense that our relationship would grow to be so strong because she told me she was unable to have kids of her own, and I was happy to fill that void she might've felt. To this day, she still works at Methodist, and we maintain contact the best we can. The morning bath ritual from Galveston did not change much, but it was at least a bit easier than it was. The big difference was that it was in something I'd describe as a giant plastic bathtub on wheels. It was still uncomfortable, but not as bad as the open flat bath table in the tub room at Shriners. Then every morning, while my wounds were being bandaged and my body creamed with Eucerin, I usually had my headphones on singing Bon Jovi out loud. The nurses laughed at my singing, but I honestly didn't care. And then the majority of my day was taken up by physical therapy, along with occasional speech therapy and recreational and social activities.

It was a week or two before Christmas; I was watching *Ghostbusters II* when a nurse came in one evening and told me I had a visitor. Her name was Amber Cooper. She was a former classmate from my fourth-grade class in Yates City and was with her mom and two sisters visiting one of her grandparents who was also a patient there at the time. Somehow she or her mother found out I was there and popped in to my room for a quick hello. That was my first time visiting with a former classmate, and I was actually as nervous and quiet as Amber was. But I was still grateful for the visit and glad they took the time to say hello and wish me well. I might have been shy, but I still appreciated being visited by folks instead of being shunned. Also, I think it was just before Christmas when I went on my first outing at the new hospital. One evening, with the help of the recreational therapists, a few patients and I were taken by wheelchair-accessible bus to the theater to see *Home Alone*. That was the first movie I saw after my burns, and it was great to get out and enjoy life outside hospitals even for just a few hours. Also, every Thursday evening the recreational therapists took a few patients and me down to the cafeteria for whatever we wanted. Pretty much every time, I opted for an overloaded salad because they had tons of topping options, but the bad part is I was still learning to feed myself, so I was still relying on being fed. It was during the first few days after arriving in Peoria when I met Don Goertzen, who was a prosthetist at Hangers Prosthetics. His first project with me was working on an adaptive tool that would allow me to feed myself. It required unscrewing the hook from the end of my arm and screwing the device in, basically replacing my hook with a fork or spoon that could rotate up or down. But eating the aforementioned salad with the new tool was still almost impossible because I was slowly learning to use it.

When Christmastime arrived, it seemed as if I was receiving stuff from everyone—Christmas cards with money, toys, even remote-controlled cars. A family member visiting my roommate Billy even let me "borrow" their Bon Jovi videos. I don't know if their intention was to give or let me borrow, but I still have one of them, and unfortunately, the other was stolen. Even a group of clowns from a local church visited and gave me an oversized plush Ninja Turtle. Just before Christmas, Don returned, but on that day, he brought along his family and a few Christmas gifts. He found out I loved Bon Jovi, so he gave me two cassette tapes and a small Boombox to play them on. I told him thank you but I already had a Boombox as well as one of the tapes. I didn't want to seem ungrateful and rude, so I told him I'll give them to my brother for Christmas. He still mentions that every now and then during prosthetic appointments and how impressed his wife was when I mentioned giving it to my brother. But actually, I felt bad they spent that money on me and I gave it to my brother.

On Christmas morning, my grandpa came with my mom to pick me up and take me to my grandparents for the day. It was my first time seeing Mom again after transferring to Methodist, and we talked a little bit during the car ride. Not only did I not have to spend the holiday in the hospital, but there was also snow on the ground and even more lightly falling. I always loved how beautiful and tranquil snow can be. My only regret is not being able to play in it as other people do. On our way there, we stopped at the new house my family moved to during my time away. Life went on while I was gone, and moving remained a fact of life for our family. Then we arrived at the familiar red house outside Alexis where my grandparents lived. My mom made sure to remind me of how Cassandra and Elric might react, because this would be the first time they saw me since my burns. The same would be true for Victor, but being older meant he better understood the scars and being burned.

Surprisingly, everyone actually reacted quite well. Joey was the most comfortable with my appearance. Because of our shared traumatic experience, we share a common bond, an understanding of each other, and he knows that inside my scars it was still me. The biggest change other than my burns was how big Elric had grown while I was away. He was barely able to speak a few words when I last saw him, and now, he could talk up a storm. My cousins Erin, Tony, and my aunt Debbie were also there for the holiday. Until Christmas of 2013, that was actually the last time all four siblings and I were under one roof. We enjoyed Christmas dinner with the usual fixings, like turkey, ham, potatoes, gravy, and one of my childhood favorites from Grandma, the scalloped corn. Then when it came time to open the presents, my grandma was Santa that year, and Joey and Tony were the elves, complete with elf costumes. I remember thinking it should have been me as the elf that year and felt left out as the others were able to go up and down the stairs at will. I got a few presents I don't remember, cookies, toys, etc., but the big one I do remember was the *Ghostbusters* firehouse headquarters. I smiled as I had the most important toy in the *Ghostbusters* lineup, which I looked forward to for months. Then I gave Victor his present, the Boombox and Bon Jovi tape. He had a look of shock on his face as if he wondered how I could possibly have gotten it for him. Then before I knew it, the sun had set, the magic had ended, and it was time for me to head back to the hospital. I didn't want the day to end. Before everyone went their separate ways, I said good-bye to my siblings and cousins. When I was back at Methodist, I remember crying a little bit because once again I would be alone. My mom promised she would visit in a few weeks and left her gold necklace around the neck of my ninja turtle as proof she would be back. Then I was alone in my room but still grateful I was able to get outside of the hospital and be with my family on my favorite holiday.

Chapter 9

As the weeks dragged on, my friendship with Diane grew stronger still. We talked and planned about day outings in Peoria for shopping, meeting her husband Bob, and even eventually staying the night at her house in Canton. The first outing with Diane was the day I met Bob. Just like Diane, we had a unique relationship over the years. I always thought of him as the dad I never had. And he knows I always had fun giving him grief; it was reciprocal. On that day, our first stop was down at the riverfront near the paddleboat. Then we went to the Peoria Zoo at Glen Oak. That was another first for me after my burns, my first zoo trip. Before I went out in public, I had no idea how I would deal with the stares and occasional questions. Sometime very early on, I somehow learned to adapt to it by acting normally and ignored it. Then we went to Toys R Us for some shopping and "spoiling." I realized I forgot the money I had saved, but Diane and Bob both told me not to worry about it. I wasn't expecting that at all, but since I had no choice, I went along with it. Keep in mind at that time I was still interested in toys I couldn't really play with and enjoy. But I ended up choosing two medium-sized toys from a toy line called Dino-Riders. I chose the *Stegosaurus* and *Diplodocus*, along with a pair of Transformers sunglasses that were actually a little too small for my head. Then we went just next door to Chuck E.

Cheese's for lunch/dinner. It had been so long since I went to one of those places that the last time I went it was still called ShowBiz Pizza Place. I had fun, but as usual, the amount of stares from other kids kind of dampened my mood by making me more self-conscious and uncomfortable. Then our last stop before we returned to the hospital was an unplanned visit to the theater. It was just around the corner from Chuck E. Cheese's, so we figured why not. I very much wanted Diane and Bob to see *Home Alone* with me because the first time around I thought it was hilarious. Then after the movie and a rather long day, we returned to Methodist. I had so much fun that day and truly appreciated my second set of parents, who never blinked an eye or thought twice about anything they did for or gave me. All of this they did without any thought of reward other than my smile and my thanks.

I was also making friends with other patients and some of their family members. First was Billy, because obviously I did share my room with him. Then there was Michael, who was paralyzed from waist down. He was a cool guy and closer to my personality and the kind of people my family knew, so that made him easy to get along with. There was another patient closer to my age, but strangely I can't recall his name. He was only a year or so older, and because of that, we shared common interests, like video games. There was an older lady patient whose grandkids came with their parents, and the four of us would hang out playing Nintendo. And last but not least were Joe Randall and his wife, Debbie. Joe was fully paralyzed and restricted to a bed. I was first introduced to Debbie, and kind of like Diane, she was a friend and a mother figure away from home. The nurses couldn't entertain me 24/7, so if Debbie was available, we would hang out in the recreational/dining area and play Monopoly or sometimes chat with Joe in his room. So all this at least made it a little less boring than the original Shriners hospital down in Galveston. There were no toys or playroom, but at least I wasn't forced to hang out in my room like at Galveston when the playroom was closed. I could come and go as I wanted.

When I wasn't busy with physical therapy or other stuff during the week, I also worked closely with a speech therapist named Bonnie Thompson. She made sure I always used my "annoying" hearing aid and worked with me on any verbal pronunciation due to my burns. She was also the person who initially got me started with computers after my burns. At first, she simply strapped a pen or pencil to my arm, and I poked and pecked at the keys. But I would eventually use my hooks and gradually get more proficient at it as I got my practice.

I fondly remember one of our morning rituals I was looking through the comics section of the newspaper. Taking a cue from a coworker, she began taping clips from Garfield on her door. I even met her daughter who at the time was taking singing and, I think, acting lessons. One day she and a few others she worked with sang a song near the nurses' station a cappella just for me. Even though I was shy and a little embarrassed from the attention all focused on me at the time, I never did forget how beautiful their voices sounded because of the love and emotion behind it and the way it made me feel all special inside.

At about the same time as that first outing, I remember watching the news one evening showing the live bombardment and attacks on Iraq during the Gulf War in operation codenamed Desert Storm. To me, it was mostly a boring news story, but it was different watching a live battle as it was happening and the fact there was also a male nurse on our floor from Iraq. Being young, I didn't understand why he was here and not an enemy. I realized he wasn't, but I still, for some reason, wasn't comfortable around him. It wasn't anything personal; I just had no experience being around somebody from the Middle East, and his accent also made it difficult to understand him most of the time. So most of the time when I needed something and he entered my room, I'd ask him to get one of the lady nurses I was more comfortable with. I'm not proud of the fact that I didn't let Abdul do his job, but at least I've grown and changed since those years. My physical therapy, speech, and daily morning treatments all still continued at their normal pace for the time being. The weekends were a respite time from the therapy, and my ritual almost every Saturday and Sunday included sitting near a window in the therapy room for hours watching, waiting, and hoping to see my mom pull into the parking garage in our new van recently acquired for us by our lawyers. Sometimes I would change it up by waiting at the elevators for seemingly hours on end. For a little amusement, sometimes I would use my wheelchair to push a trash can directly in front of the elevator doors. I had nothing else to do but sit and wait anyway, so why not have a little fun? To break up some of the monotony, I would sometimes go outside with staff to enjoy some fresh air, drive my wheelchair around in the snow, or watch the birds on their feeders. I don't remember exactly when, but sometime around early spring, my roommate Billy was allowed to go home. This meant I had the room to myself, and from then on, for whatever reason, the staff decided to keep it that way.

It was just sometime around March 1991 when I went back down to Galveston for my first checkup. This time, my mom and Joey would be flying down with me. As a matter of fact, that would be the only time we flew together until many years later. As usual, I enjoyed my now traditional in-flight ginger ale while we played with Hot Wheels to keep us occupied during the flight. When we arrived, the Shriners were already there waiting. I was always apprehensive after landing in Houston. The Shriners would take over, and it was almost like an added loss of control. It was like the Shriners symbolized all the pain that might await me. They were the deliverers so to speak. Seeing the Shriners back then, I liken it to a new prisoner approaching the guards and officers who would escort him to prison. I didn't hate them, but I didn't have the sense of appreciation for them that I have now. From there, the only destination was the hospital, and I couldn't change that fact. I tried to delay our arrival and extend our time by asking to stop for a drink, but it didn't last. Eventually, I had to face the music. After arriving, almost immediately I was given a bath despite my protests that I already had one that morning. Meanwhile, my mom and Joey checked into a nearby hotel. I don't recall how long that stay was, but it set the stage for what future checkups would be like. The therapists evaluated my progress or sometimes loss of progress due to skin tightening and contracting—seeing how my wounds and scars were healing, taking photos, talking to psychologists, evaluating for possible surgeries, and the list goes on. Fortunately, that time I was able to go back to Peoria without having any surgeries done. When I landed at Peoria Airport, Bob Wells was there waiting for me. I had not seen him in at least a month or so, and that was my first time I had seen him with his beard shaved off. Upon seeing him, I had no clue that he was, but as he talked to me, he seemed to know me better than I knew him, and I realized he was indeed Bob.

I was back at Methodist in Peoria and glad I didn't have to face any surgeries. But in the weeks ahead, I faced new problems. There always seemed to be something new to deal with, whether it was a new wound on my body or whatever the case may be. There was never a dull moment, and I don't remember exactly what was happening, but my skin seemed to be reacting to something, and later on that spring, the nurses and doctors were taking the JOBST off of my limbs, which left them exposed, uncovered, and unprotected. I didn't like this feeling, and even today, all four limbs are always covered with socks. And because of this, I was also unable to wear my upper prosthetics very much if at all, further limiting the already-slow learning progress of using and adapting to them. But definitely, the most painful part of my daily schedule at that time was the physical therapy. For the most part, it was tolerable and not too bad. But every day when the therapist started to bend my right elbow, the pain was excruciating. The way my right elbow is now, it's permanently fused at a ninety-degree angle with only a few degrees movement. It cannot be fixed without major surgery requiring a stainless-steel contraption that would slowly bend it over six to nine months. I don't remember if my elbow was fused back then, but it barely budged while the therapist pushed and pulled with all her strength. As she did this, I cried in pain every time, and I'm not ashamed to admit it. Even when I was down in Galveston therapy with Merilyn or any other therapist, it never hurt as much as that, and part of me thought something wasn't right. Just about every morning when I went into the therapy room at Methodist, I would try to somehow get out of it sometimes by crying, but I usually feigned sickness by feeling like I was going to throw up. When I think about it, my fear of the pain was probably a valid reason for that sick feeling. Somebody would then grab a bucket to puke in, and nevertheless, anything short of actual death, the torture always continued. I also must mention that at some point during the spring of '91 was the first mention of any scoliosis. It started off simply as nurses and therapists telling me to stop crossing my legs, but I shrugged it off and honestly did not see any harm in it, and if I knew then what I know now, I would have done much more to keep the scoliosis from worsening. The scoliosis unfortunately is another subject I'll discuss in greater detail in the next book, because it didn't begin to affect me until many years later.

I grew increasingly attached to Diane as time went on. Eventually, I did go to her house for an overnight stay a few times. And almost every time, those overnight stays were accompanied with a shopping trip, movie rentals, and good nonhospital food. Then on Sunday, it would be time for us to head back to Methodist. Before the Spring Thaw set in that year, Diane and a few nurses took Michael and me to the Ice Capades at the Peoria Civic Center. Michael admittedly looked forward to seeing Barbie on Ice, while I was there to see the Simpsons part of the show. Prior to the event, the Bart Simpson costumed character visited our floor of the hospital, and I got a picture with him, cool man. That was an early example of one of the very few perks of being severely burned. As I said before, it was those special events and occasions that made dealing with the hardships easier; they were just a small tradeoff for the everyday things I would miss out on or never get to experience. So when people say, "Oh, you're so lucky," they should realize they are too. An able-bodied person is lucky every day because they can look forward to so many things they can easily do that I'll never get to do or miss out on entirely. Perks are short-lived and are few between, but an able body is for a lifetime. Or when anyone says to me something for example "you're not the one who has to wash the dishes, etc.", I'd pay anything to be able to. Don't get me wrong though, I'm not suggesting anyone who is disabled, paralyzed, etc. or whatever the case may be that we have nothing to be grateful or thankful for. Just that you should count your blessings and be grateful for even the simplest things that the able bodied take for granted every day.

I also kept up with my weekend routine of staring out the window and hanging out near the elevator in hope of my family visiting. On a few occasions, my aunt Leslie visited, bringing my cousin Chad and Samantha with her. My cousin Lea Ann also visited a few times with her friend tagging along. My Aunt Lisa even took the time to visit a few times. Though I can still remember my cousin Nick's initial reaction during the first visit. He was very quiet and barely uttered a word the entire time, but on the next visit he seemed like a different kid entirely. The first time around he seemed to distance himself like he didn't know who I was and then during his next visit did a complete flip as if I wasn't burned at all. Some people just don't know to react and completely freeze up but Nick got over it pretty quickly. It was about early April just after returning from Galveston when my mom found out she was pregnant with her sixth. I just couldn't believe I would have yet another sibling. I thought that having more kids had ended four years before then. I spent the night at home with my family at least once during this period. My mom didn't have a lot of time and money for multiple trips and overnight stays at that time, especially with my new sibling coming. There was one particular weekend when my family visited we went down to the hospital gift shop just for a chance to get off my floor. On that day, something happened to me that hasn't occurred since then. I left the gift shop and zoomed around the corner down a small hallway. I had zoomed off while my family was still in the shop, and I was quickly turning around to go back, but as I turned around, a young black boy about Joey's age jumped from around the corner, held up his hands, and yelled out "Rawr" with an ugly look on his face. He immediately ran off afterward, but nobody else was around to see it happen. I was angry and frustrated that I couldn't get out of my wheelchair, chase him down, and teach him a lesson. Those feelings of frustration would be a part of my life from then on, but that was the only time I was confronted so aggressively by a total stranger, and he was so young. A few weeks after Mom told me about being pregnant again, my family visited me in the hospital, and we went to the Peoria Zoo and Toys R Us just for the day. Joey realized he had been there before with his kindergarten class from Yates City. But it didn't matter to me either way because I was just glad to get out of the hospital for a few hours. That day was also one of those rare occasions when my mom actually had and was willing to spend a few bucks on something a little more extravagant. For a while, I had my sights set on the big *Tyrannosaurus rex* from the Dino-Riders toy line. But on that day, none were in stock, and I got the next best thing. The *T. rex* might have been my first choice, but the one I got was actually much bigger. Mom bought me a huge *Brontosaurus* Dino-Rider set. Even today, I'm pretty sure that thing remains the biggest toy version ever produced of a *Brontosaurus*. But those happier days were not going to last. I was still dealing with skin problems and most likely faced possible surgical reconstruction.

The first anniversary of my burns on April 19 had come and gone that first year with barely a blink. It was middle afternoon one day late May when I finally received the news I had been dreading and yet knew it was coming. Diane and a social worker named Sue told me that everything was all set up and I was heading back down to Galveston and almost definitely would expect more surgeries. I had become comfortable during my time at Methodist and not only hated this disruption of my sense of control, but of course, I also feared the impending surgeries and pain that went along with them. I cried as I pleaded not to go even though I knew it would do no good. A dark cloud had been cast over the rest of that day and would remain there until I left. That weekend, Diane and her husband, Bob, took me out on a day shopping trip in an attempt to ease my tension before I left. I don't know why I remember such materialistic things, but they cheered me up and helped to brighten my mood on the gloomiest days, but on that day, I ended up getting yet another toy I couldn't manipulate, the official *Teenage Mutant Ninja Turtle* party wagon attack van. It was a cool toy, and I still get nostalgic when I think about those early toys and a shame I don't have it anymore. The staff of 4 Hamilton had a going-away party for me just before I left. There was a good-bye cake with a red fern on it (I was reading *Where the Red Fern Grows*), a banner, and cards from everybody who was there to wish me well until I returned. Diane came with me to the airport, where I met up with my mom for my flight. It was official; there was no turning back from that point. I didn't know how long I'd be gone. Only that I knew a surgery was pretty much inevitable. And that small detail just made me feel powerless, not unlike how my youngest brother, Elric, felt while he was crying when Mom left him behind at the airport. I knew exactly how he felt. Once again, he too was watching Mom leave as I did so many times before. Finally, one of the last things Diane said to me before I boarded was that I could call her anytime I needed as she quickly wrote her phone number on my orange neon hat. Before I knew it, the plane was on the runway taking off, and I was once again on my way to Galveston.

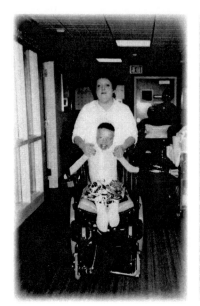
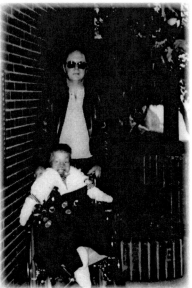

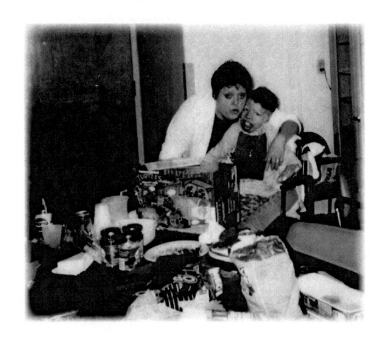

Chapter 10

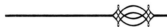

It was June of 1991, and I was back at Shriners in Galveston for a round of inevitable surgeries. I hated the surgical and healing process that followed afterward, especially during those early days and that particular summer. Every time I went under the knife, it felt like I was reset, as if I had to do everything all over again to get back to the quality of life I enjoyed before each surgery. Even though my mom had come with me, she was already gone before I had my first one. Though she visited once that summer during a checkup with Joey, I wouldn't see her again until my birthday in October. I don't remember how many I had nor what each individual surgery was for, but I do remember some of the details from a few of them and the accompanying healing processes. That round of surgeries wasn't much different than the year before except for the fact that I was no longer bedridden and I had my power wheelchair with me. The wheelchair would at least help alleviate my boredom instead of sitting in one place for hours without end. I can't honestly say which surgery came first, but I think one of the earlier procedures was another neck release. The neck release would prevent further skin contracting and allow me to turn and tilt my head farther. After the surgery, I was restricted to a bed for a week minimum while my neck healed. During that time, for a few days, I ate very little to almost no food.

That's just how my after-surgery routine was back then. Because the surgery was meant to prevent constricting, my neck was tilted back as far as it could until the time came to remove the bandages. In the meantime, my bed was turned around backward so I could watch TV albeit I had to watch it upside down. Still, I'd rather watch it upside down than not at all. And it wouldn't be that last time either.

My initial stay the year before was spent in the ward for newly burned patients on the same floor, but on the other side of the hospital. On the new side, it was a mostly different nursing staff, and it had somewhat relaxed restrictions regarding visitors and infection control. A big difference was I no longer used the tub room on the other side. The new ward unfortunately lacked some of the modern equipment the other room had, and thus, the baths were just as unpleasant as they were at the other tub room. Everything else from before, including child life therapists, remained basically the same as before, except now I was half the distance to the playroom. Even though the nursing staff was mostly new to me, there was a very small few that for whatever reason seemed to hold a grudge toward me. I have always wondered if perhaps the same nurse from the previous summer who had hit me possibly told a few others. Who knows. But one older black female nurse would stand out above the rest with her misguided angst, and back then when it happened, I never did tell anyone about such things. I was eleven, alone, and I wouldn't have family to visit or back me up the entire summer. Back then, I wasn't aware of any options I had of dealing with it, so I kept it to myself. Gene was still a nurse on this floor too, so at least I had him around. But there was a male nurse I hadn't met prior named Mr. Loflin. He wasn't mean or anything, but his personality and manner was just too much for me. The best way I could describe him was a combination of a marine drill sergeant and the classic Looney Tunes character Foghorn Leghorn the chicken, whom I didn't like either. Mr. Loflin was also mentioned in another book titled *Riley* written by his mom Lee Merril Boyd. Maybe he was too rough, gruff, and Southern for me because after all I'm a northern Yankee from Illinois, but in her book, it seems she too was sometimes overwhelmed by his personality. One of the most special friendships I made that summer was with somebody not even on the hospital staff. She was a fellow patient. Her name was Crystal Rodriguez. She was then five years old and had been shot in the leg during the previous riots in Panama. She would hang out in my room and watch cartoons or try to sneak into my candy stash. She always wanted to play, and in a way, she was like the little sister away from home. She was fun to be around and play with but at other times could be annoying just like a sibling.

I kept in touch with Diane via phone, and she also mailed me care packages filled with my favorite candies and a can or two of SpaghettiOs for those days when I was bored with hospital food. Whenever the playroom was open and I was able to go, Crystal and I were usually there playing. Luckily, by then, I had finally managed to use both arms for playing video games. When I was fortunate enough to have them on consistently, it was a step up from doing nothing and learning how to adapt to them. Learning to play video games with my prosthetics was actually easy because prior to being burned, I never had my own Nintendo or a Gameboy. I had asked for a Nintendo before my burns, but it was just too much to ask for back then. My surgeries continued relentlessly though. Almost as soon as I had healed from one surgery, I was back under the knife again. But the surgeries that summer for some reason had a big difference than almost all that came before. Almost every surgery, I was still awake as I went into the operating room, and some type of aerosol was sprayed up my nose, and a huge breathing tube was inserted in my nose all while I was awake. This was one of the scariest and most painful processes I ever went through more than once. Even though it was somewhat fast, I couldn't breathe the entire time it was being inserted. It was like suffocation, and I couldn't get away from it. Only when it was done did I succumb to the effects of the anesthesia. To be honest, that part of the surgery by itself was a big reason I feared them. If they had opted to do it differently, I probably wouldn't have feared future surgeries so much. The traumatic memory of the insertion stuck with me; thus, it was a subconscious fear each and every time even after they no longer did it that way.

Not only was I dealing with surgeries, healing, accompanying therapy, and the necessary garments, but further things being done made it feel like I was a guinea pig. It seemed almost weekly even sometimes daily that some unknown technician or specialist would come into my room with this pencil-shaped medical tool. But instead of a pink eraser on the end, it had a sharp round edge like a mini cookie cutter. This end was jabbed into my skin in order to pull out tissue samples. As to why the samples were needed, I had no idea. I couldn't help but think sometimes that just maybe somebody was indeed trying to make my time there as difficult as possible. But every time it was done, I was angry, because I just could not see the logic of something that seemed so barbaric to me. I remember thinking to myself, *Stab that thing in your arm and see how much you like it.* I also had to deal with surgical staples and their removal. Most of the time, it wasn't too bad when they were removed, but there was also a few rare occasions where they had to insert staples while I was not in surgery and awake. Inserting a staple is way different than its removal and obviously more painful. Just imagine using a normal office stapler on yourself, and that is basically an accurate description of what it felt like. Furthermore, the whole summer, I had to constantly deal with the heat. Surprisingly, there was no air conditioning in this hospital, so I very much needed the aid of a fan to keep cool enough. But my fan was constantly being taken away for use by the lab technicians, or so I was told. That was another thing that didn't make much sense to me for multiple reasons. After all, since it was Texas, things could get very hot down there, so why wasn't there any other fans available in the entire hospital, and why they couldn't possibly bring their own? And most of all, I was a severe burn survivor unable to sweat, thus I overheat very easily, so you think my medical needs and comfort would have been a higher priority.

I was looking forward to the Fourth of July because Catherine promised to take me out that night for pizza at her house and then see the fireworks at the beach. I missed the holiday the previous year, because obviously I was still restricted to a bed. I didn't want to miss out two years in a row, so when I found out from a nurse that I had a surgery scheduled just before the holiday, I was crying and somewhat pissed off. Enough already. Give me a break long enough to enjoy the holiday and then let the torture resume. Didn't I deserve that small request? I called Diane and told her what was up, and I don't remember exactly who talked to whom, but the surgery was rescheduled until after the holiday. This small victory brightened my mood, and I had a great night out with Catherine. She took me to her place for pizza, then later on, she drove me to the top of a parking deck near the hospital to watch the fireworks. Those things might not seem like a big deal, but the relationships I've had over the years with people like Catherine and the kindness they've shown simply made me feel special inside and are just another example of how the joy from even the little things helped distract me from the pain and everyday difficulties.

One of the more painful surgeries that summer involved my chest. I don't remember exactly what the procedure was for, but the healing process afterward was torture in itself. Every morning and evening involved changing a bandage on my chest and thoroughly cleaning it with a solution that had salt in it. That stuff stung like hell mostly because the wound surface was so large. It was during one of those evening treatments when the aforementioned black nurse said something to me that I won't forget. I always did my best to be nice to her and the others. I had manners, I never talked back, I didn't cuss, and I did as I was told. But that evening in front of the other nurses, while cleaning my chest wound, she stuck a $100 bill down her bra and said, "If you grab it, you can have it." I told her I don't have my arm on anyway, and I'm not that kind of kid. She then said, "Yeah, you are, and you know it." There was also more than one occasion when she and other nurses allowed Crystal into my room during more "private" moments like when I was using a handheld urinal or anything nude. The nurse was like, "It's nothing she hasn't seen before," but that didn't make it all right. That black nurse should consider herself very lucky I don't remember her name and the fact that I never did officially report anything. How could I? The other nurses were right there when she said that and were laughing like nothing was wrong. This made me feel powerless, like I had nobody on my side, and if I did say something, no good could have come from it. I still don't understand what I did to possibly merit all the hate she aimed at me.

Sometime around midsummer, one of the head female nurses (unfortunately, I don't remember her name) took me out for a day trip with her family to Lone Star Flight Museum. I remember meeting her daughter Elizabeth and realized I liked the name. I later suggested the name to Mom for my yet unborn sister, and it stuck. The museum was a cool outing. It had still operating war planes from WWII in the collection. Though back then I wasn't as much into history and aircraft as I am now. Airplanes were cool to me then, but I lacked the awe, wonder, and respect an older person might have for them. One of the other surgeries I remember toward the middle to late summer was an attempt to straighten my right elbow. My therapist Merilyn explained to me prior to the surgery that when I awoke from surgery, my right arm would be in a machine that would slowly bend it back and forth. When I awoke afterward, I didn't feel my arm moving and realized there was no machine. I don't remember why, but for whatever reason, it didn't go as planned, and my right elbow today remains very much the same as it was then. I know there were a few more here and there, but the only other surgery I can remember was another axilla release under my arms. That surgery was difficult due to the fact that afterward I still had to endure these very uncomfortable airplane splints. The splints were meant to prevent my arms contracting back down. And I was forced to wear them at night for a few months.

Sometime around midsummer, I must admit I had a short-lived breakdown in the middle of the night. It happened sometime after the surgery on my chest. For whatever reason, that night I was so uncomfortable, possibly from heat or a combination of things. I became so frustrated and angry that I just started yelling and screaming. I was frustrated and pissed off at anyone and everything, and I don't fully remember why, nor did I ever express myself like that before or since then. One of the nurses entered my room and said, "Shut up, everyone is sleeping." A patient crying from pain at random hours was nothing new, but the outburst I had that night was so unlike me. Like I said, I don't remember what made me explode that night, but whatever reason it was, I guess I just had to let it out. Even the strongest individuals have their moments when they feel overwhelmed like they can't take it anymore.

Toward late summer, Bonnie Bishop introduced me to a neighbor of hers who was in the coast guard. I don't remember his name, but he visited with me and taught me all sorts of things about working on a ship. He told me about how port meant left and starboard meant right. And that the bow refers to the front and the stern was the rear of a boat. He even explained how the navigation lights left and right were red and green respectively. He was even able to take me out for a short stroll in my wheelchair just behind the hospital one day when the clouds unleashed a flood of rain. We were getting absolutely drenched until we took shelter in a building at the shrimp boat docks in the area behind the hospital. Even though we had been soaked, the rain didn't bother me. And it gave us time to hang out longer at the dock till the rain stopped. Plus it was kind of neat seeing the shrimp boats as they left to harvest their bounties. It wasn't long after that when Merilyn took me out for a day trip. That day, I met her husband, Carl, who was a helicopter mechanic working at Galveston Airport. He got permission for me to go out onto the tarmac and see the helicopters up-close. I was even allowed to sit in one. After the airport, we went to Walmart, and I still remember I chose a Lego coast guard set, which I later showed to Bonnie's neighbor. Merilyn also took to me her house by Galveston Lake, and Carl showed me his Matchbox car collection and his computer games. Merilyn later told me, "What was interesting was that you seemed much more excited about shopping for toys/games at Walmart and playing computer games with Carl at our apartment! It was that excitement and talent that impressed Carl." And Carl also commented to Merilyn, "That he could see the real little boy in there, despite your appearance and horrific experiences." Yeah, toys and video games were fun, and I seemed somewhat focused on them back then, but I remember how cool it was when Carl told me the Huey helicopter I saw up-close on the tarmac that day had served over in the Persian Gulf during Desert Storm.

Toward the end of summer just a few weeks before I returned home, I remember one of my worst evenings. To put it short, I was still having problems going to the bathroom, and that night was spent flushing my system with another enema, but this one seemed to be extra strong. Proof being the next day in the therapy room, even Crystal could tell something wasn't right. She asked Ms. Josey, the therapy technician, "What's wrong with Caper?" Ms. Josey then told her I was sick, and that was the truth—I truly felt like crap. That was probably the last bad day before I returned home. Crystal had her own troubles too. Not long after that, she finally had the rod removed from her leg. I was in the therapy room with her on the day her surgeon entered the room. She looked up, and without blinking, she immediately started crying. I sympathized with her, but I knew it was in her best interest and she would soon be walking again.

In late September, it was decided that Crystal and I would celebrate our birthdays on the same day with a birthday party in the playroom. I don't remember the date of Crystal's birthday, but mine was on October 4, and I would be home by then. The party had the usual fun stuff, like clowns, balloons, cake, ice cream, candy, and of course, the birthday presents. I don't remember what Crystal asked for and received, but prior to the party, I described to Catherine I wanted a Fast Traxx RC car. I told her it was like a tank. She told the Shriners, who picked it up, and I opened it, and it was a tank. I was like oops I must have confused you with what I was asking for. The Fast Traxx wasn't a tank, but it had treads like one. I told them the tank was fine, and I didn't want to seem disappointed or ungrateful, but one of the Shriners who bought it said he knew what I was talking about because it had been near the tank. Keep in mind at the time there were very few things I could play with. So far up to that point, it had just been Legos and Nintendo. Very soon, within a day or two after the party, I was given the Fast Traxx I wanted. I had RC cars in the past, but I was unable to play with them, and this one was also faster. I quickly learned how to operate it and raced it down the hallway while Crystal watched. It was two birds with one stone. I had a new way to play with something, and I was further learning how to use and adapt to my prosthesis. My overall mood and joy in those few short days before I returned home had skyrocketed, and I couldn't wait to return to everyone at Methodist again.

On the morning of my flight back home, I went by Crystal's room to peek in and said good-bye one last time while she was still sleeping. I still think about her sometimes, and I haven't seen her since then, and I hope she is doing well. Merilyn accompanied me yet again on this trip, but this time would not be in Peoria for an extended stay. Almost on the very same day I returned, the annual Methodist Rehabilitation Ceremony was held at the atrium building across the street from the hospital. It was a way of recognizing patients, therapists, and staff of the rehab floor of their achievements and hard work. Even I received a small plaque, but I'll admit, back then, I felt I didn't deserve one because of all the crying I had done during those painful therapy sessions, and in my opinion, at the time, I didn't yet have the huge success and comeback stories of other patients. There were also food and drinks, and I also got to say hello to a few patients who had went home during my time at Methodist. But most of all, I was just glad to be home, and it almost seemed like the ceremony was a welcome-home party held just for me. I knew it wasn't, but it was still nice to have a party and see everyone again after my long and difficult summer down in Galveston.

It seemed like my twelfth birthday came almost immediately after the rehab awards. My mom told me she wasn't going to be able to make it, unfortunately, but the huge party the staff held for me helped make up for it. Just like my going-away party months earlier, this one had a banner, cake, snacks, and last but not least, birthday presents. After I blew out the candles on the cake, I made a spur-of-the-moment decision influenced by *America's Funniest Home Videos*, and I slammed my face down into the cake. Those cakes always had too much sugar, but I still enjoyed the "cake face" moment. Strangely, I only remember one present from that birthday, and it was from Diane and Bob. It was a Tyco Turbo Train. It was basically a slot car but with the shell of a train instead of a car. It was set up for me on one of the therapy mat tables. But the day wasn't all fun and games. I had an appointment to get my eyes looked at that afternoon. Diane told me they were going to put a drop in my eyes that would make my vision blurry for a few hours afterward. This kind of bummed my evening, but after I was given the drops and it was finished, I never really did notice any difference in my vision, so no harm, no foul.

The final surprise that day was when my mom and siblings showed up that evening. I hadn't seen any of them for months, and the first thing I did was show Joey my Turbo Train. We tried racing them, but he was better at it, and even he had trouble keeping them on the track while the railcars were connected to the engines, so we took them off. All in all, the first few days of being back home in Illinois at Methodist were great, and I was settling back into my comfortable routine, but more changes were coming.

Chapter 11

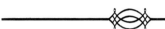

By the fall of '91, I was wearing my upper prosthesis pretty much all day. My lower prosthesis required the assistance of therapists for walking, but I also wore them an hour or so a day, slowly increasing my pressure tolerance. The days were about the same as before, but now I was becoming more active because there were more things I was capable of doing. I was playing with Legos during some of my occupational therapy sessions. I was quickly adapting more to using them every day. Because of my hearing, Bonnie thought my TV should have closed captioning. Back then, it required a separate decoder box. I was actually not looking forward to the annoying device, but once I started using it, I ended up preferring the device. To this day, I still will not watch a show or movie without closed captioning or subtitles. I simply miss too much of the dialogue without it. I can hear it but can't understand much of what I hear. There was one memorable weekend I went shopping with Diane that sparked a new interest for me. So far I had Legos, Nintendo, and my Fast Traxx apart from TV and movies to keep me occupied. But on that particular day, Diane bought me a few packs of Micro Machines and their respective highways and byways city set. I had liked them before, but their small size made it easy for me to manipulate and play with them. It was a "eureka, aha" moment. I finally had something I could play with and collect. The late months of '91, my collection grew rapidly, and I never did stop collecting them until they ended production many years later.

By the fall season of '91, I had been out of school for over a year and missed my entire fifth grade year. So to try and keep my education on track, the first big change early that fall was tutoring. I was introduced to several local teachers over the course of a few days so I could determine who I was comfortable with and who I would prefer being my tutor. I chose Edie as my tutor mainly for the reason she told me we could make a volcano. Since I did like dinosaurs, volcanoes sort of fell into that realm of interest, and it was what clinched the decision for me. My daytime routine remained the same with physical therapy and the usual stuff, and then Edie would come in for a few hours in the evening. Though I'll be honest in the earlier sessions, we seemed to do more talking about things than anything else. We got along fine, and gradually, she did push the talking aside to get into the learning. I don't remember how long the tutoring continued, but I do know how it ended. It was a Friday, and after my tutoring, I was once again going to Diane's house for the weekend. I was anxious and excited to go. Keep in mind when you have been in the hospital for over a year, you savor every chance you get outside those walls. So while she was instructing me on something that session, I excitedly said something like, "Okay, I got it, I got it," trying to get her to move on. I meant no offense at all; I was just overly excited for my weekend, but Edie snapped. I don't remember her exact words, but she stormed out, and I sat there feeling conflicted and dumbfounded. I didn't mean to anger or hurt her feelings, but on the other hand, I was free to leave for the weekend. Diane entered my room and asked me, "What was that all about?" I explained to her what happened, and she didn't blame me at all. I mean really, I was no different than any kid ready to leave school for the day, except I was stuck where I was for days on end. So *who* could blame me?

That fall there were actually only two difficult things I remember I dealt with. The first was the day I suffered a bladder infection. I woke up one morning with a sharp pain below my stomach that just wouldn't go away. I got up and into my wheelchair, and the pain was still throbbing constantly. I wanted to get back into bed and try to sleep it away. Meanwhile, Diane and the head nurse were trying to figure out what might be wrong. They determined I had a bladder infection and I needed to drink more water. Diane said I had to cut back on the sodas and drink more water. If it meant avoiding that pain again, it was fine by me. To this day, I always try to drink enough water, and I haven't had another bladder infection ever since then.

The other event was a difficult challenge of a different kind. I had talked a few times with my lawyers over the past year. But the day came when I had a day-long interview session with a judge, my lawyers, and I assume the attorneys for McCabe Scrap Iron. My mom was in the room as well as Diane, and I think a few others, but my focus was on answering the difficult questions I faced. When we started, I was told to tell the truth and asked if I knew the difference between right and wrong. The day was long and tedious, and I felt like a murder suspect being interrogated by detectives who hoped I would crack under the pressure and confess. They asked specific questions, including how I got in, what I saw and did inside, and how I broke the gas pump. One of the final questions I remember being asked was if I knew what a propane tank was and if I knew that there was one on the property. I gave a fully honest answer to that question at that time—no. I had no clue what a propane tank was, nor did I know about the tank on the property. I later asked Diane what a propane tank was, and she explained it for me. My mom was there and heard every question given and answer I gave them. I felt so guilty and shameful when I left the conference room that day. What made it worse and seemed to intensify my feelings of guilt was the look on my mom's face. It seemed like she knew the truth and was ashamed of me also. I asked Joey if he was interviewed the same day I was, because I don't remember. I'm pretty sure he was, because later that evening we got a moment alone by ourselves in the therapy room and we talked about all the questions and the pressure. We shared the same sentiments about how we felt about the questions and the situation. I don't recall the exact words, but it was something along the lines of they know we were hiding the truth and/or we knew more than we were saying. But the explosion and the guilt were too fresh and too strong for us to move on yet.

Before I knew it, Halloween had passed, and the holidays had arrived again. I spent Thanksgiving at Diane's that year. It was my first Thanksgiving outside a hospital, and it was fully complete with all the traditional fixings, of course, turkey, deviled eggs, cranberry sauce, potatoes, and real gravy. Hospital food tended to get boring real fast, so every meal outside the hospital was a luxurious treat in my opinion.

A few weeks before Elizabeth was born, my mom told me she would call as soon as the day had come but wouldn't be able to visit again until after then. I never did get the call, and it was almost Christmas when I saw Elizabeth the first time. But the rest of the year until Christmas was mostly uneventful. The entire rehab floor was involved in a secret Santa gift exchange thing. Everyone had stockings with their names on them, including mine, and random people would leave gifts for whoever they chose. Mine ended up being full of Micro Machines packs. For the actual holiday, I went to Diane's the day before Christmas Eve and had a small party with her brother Alan and his family. Diane amazingly was the youngest of twelve siblings, and Alan was whom I knew and got along with most. I picked on him almost as much as I did Bob. Later that night, Bob and Diane took me up to Galesburg so I could spend the entire holiday at home with my family. We usually went to their house, but with my wheelchair and new sister, I guess it was easier to have them visit us, and so Grandma and Grandpa came by that evening and watched us open our presents they gave us. I just can't emphasize how grateful I am to have such great grandparents who never missed my birthday or Christmas. Aside from the gifts what was important is that they played an active role as grandparents who enjoyed spending time and even spoiling us. They were always selfless and gave without any thought of reward except our love. Biologically my grandparents were related only to my older brother and me and yet they still loved and treated us all equally. Anyhow, that year, at the top of my wish list was a Super Nintendo. I wasn't disappointed, and after my grandparents went home, we immediately hooked it up to the TV and started playing. Joey and I were the oldest and most video game coordinated, so obviously, we were the best. Victor was still in Arizona with our aunt Debbie at the time, so he wasn't there that year. Compared to how bad things seemed that summer, the year was ending on a high note. Life was a roller coaster with its ups and downs of good and bad moments. At that point in time, I had nothing to complain about. I was pain-free and torture-free and still had things to look forward to in the near future.

On Christmas Day, we went to the house of Kirk's grandmother in Knoxville for a Christmas party with their family. I actually liked her and her house before my burns, but it wasn't exactly wheelchair-friendly. She had a fully furnished basement with functioning kitchens and bathrooms on both floors. But of course, whichever floor I was on would be where I stayed. Joey and I played with our newest RC cars in the back room even though the signals interfered with each other, making the control rather erratic. I remember Kirk's stepmom always bought us gifts we could play with together. Back in 1988, we got G.I. Joe, and in 1989, she bought us Matchbox and Hot Wheels cars. This year, it was RC cars, and that was also the last time I was at his grandmother's house and my final holiday with Kirk's family.

Not long after the holiday season in 1991, I started going to school while still in the hospital. Early on, I was very apprehensive about going back to school and how I would handle things. Who would help me with all the stuff I needed help with? Things like getting books, going from class to class, lunchtime, and last but not least, my "personal" needs. And what about dealing with being around so many kids and the stares and questions? Prior to my first day, I visited Charles A. Lindbergh Middle School, and to get me somewhat acquainted, I was given a tour of the school and met some of the faculty and students. But the main focus was to teach the school therapists and personal attendants about my therapy and daily needs. I should point out that Lindbergh Middle School had regular classrooms along with separate classrooms and staff specifically for students with physical and mental disabilities. On the day I visited, I got more attention than I was used to. I was shy before my burns, but even more so afterward, thus all those new faces gathered around me was a little overwhelming. My hearing loss is a big reason for that and still is a factor in my social life today. But overall, the students and staff at Lindbergh made me feel welcome, and for the most part in terms of teasing and bullying or excessive annoyance due to stares or whatever, I actually had no trouble from anyone during my three years I was there.

Chapter 12

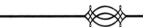

It seemed like it would never arrive, but on February 8, 1992, the day I had waited for almost two years had finally come. I was going home! The day before I left for home, I returned from school to the hospital only to be swarmed by reporters and cameras when I was led into the conference room. The amount of lights and cameras flashing was so intense I literally could barely see anyone behind the glare. I felt like a deer frozen in the headlights. The glare was so bad they could have pointed a hunting rifle at me and I would not have seen it, so thank God I wasn't a deer, eh. The local television stations were covering my story, as well as a few newspapers. The headline in the *Peoria Journal Star* article written by Phil Luciano was "'Miracle' Boy Finally Goes Home." The main message of the article was about going home after almost two years of surgeries and treatment. The article mentions me showing off my hand-to-eye coordination by demonstrating my Nintendo skills and operating my RC truck. "As nurses scurried away from the whizzing toy, one said with a smile, 'Needless to say, Caper has brought life here.'" The friendships and care I received at Methodist, I'll never forget. And Diane Wells, who was my mom away from home, still remained a big part of my life over the years, as did her husband, Bob. The next morning, I was on my way home, albeit in the back of a medical transport rig. It honestly wasn't how I pictured going home, but things don't always go how I plan or picture it. Ironically, I left the hospital the same way I entered almost two years prior, on a patient gurney in the back of an ambulance. My power chair for the time being had to stay at school until a ramp was installed at my house in Monmouth, Illinois. When I arrived home, the person transporting me asked my mom if she wanted me transferred to my bed. Already, I felt a loss of control and freedom, and in my head, I was thinking I didn't get out of the hospital today just so I could be bedridden at home and waiting for whatever treatment might be. Thankfully, it wasn't like that, and aside from going over a few medical details with my mom and the fact that Western Illinois Home Health Care staff also had training prior to my coming home, it all went smoothly.

One of the most difficult things about those days was getting up early for school. Every school day, my home nurse arrived, and I was showered and dressed starting at 5:00 a.m. The ride to school was a little over fifty miles one way. From my house, the ride to school began when a Monmouth handicap van took me to Galesburg, where we waited for, and I was transferred to a small bus with about five students all headed for three different schools in Peoria. Every morning for almost the entire ride from Monmouth to Peoria, I would lay my head down on my hearing aid box I placed on my lapboard across the armrests of my chair. It wasn't perfect sleep, but it was better than nothing, and on more than one occasion, I was still asleep when I arrived at school. The ride home was a little different. Sometimes I would nap on the ride back, but eventually that spring, I started reading books at a fast pace. I was reading lots of classic books like *White Fang, Call of the Wild, Black Stallion, The Bear,* and *Where the Red Fern Grows.* I actually earned a top ten reader award during my first two years at Lindbergh. Never in my school life had I been more proud of an educational accomplishment. It was a nice change to be acknowledged at school for once.

I gradually adjusted to life at school and got used to the staff and students. Mr. Simpson was one of the caretakers at school, and I always liked the guy. One day after showing him my newest gadget/toy, he told me to show my teacher Mrs. Rynearson. I was reluctant at first, but he had my back, so I began to show her my new "pen," and as she looked right at it, I pulled the trigger and a small burst of water shot out the top end. It was the new Super Soaker pen. Mr. Simpson was laughing his ass off, while Mrs. R just gave me that look of surprise and "Boys will be boys." Indeed, that was true, because later that same day, I was shooting small bursts straight up over the head of a classmate during a study period. She kept looking up at the ceiling and had no clue what was going on. I hid my laughter as best I could and continued doing it until it was empty, and she never suspected a thing. I still smile thinking about that one. After lunch most days, I would race my wheelchair around outside during recess, just joking with some of the girls by playfully scaring them. Obviously, I know better now, but back then, I guess it was my way of flirting and getting attention from them. I just didn't know how to act properly around them. But eventually, I stopped when I teased with the wrong girl who yelled at me to back off. I didn't mean any harm, but she took it personally. That incident affected my behavior from then on, and I changed it as a result.

Things at home were fine for a few short months during the spring. One of the biggest physical accomplishments was actually discovered by accident. One day during my ride home from school, somehow I managed to learn how to lift myself up in my wheelchair and reposition without asking somebody to help. This might seem like no big deal, but it really was. Up to that point, I was still asking for help to be pulled up in my chair whenever I needed it, which was actually quite often. But now, I was able to do it myself, and I took another step forward to independence. It was one less thing I had to rely on others to do for me. Diane and Bob maintained contact with me from the very beginning. Every few weeks or so, they would drive to my house in Monmouth and take me to Galesburg for lunch and a little bit of shopping. On other occasions, she would pick me up, and I'd go to her house for a weekend, which in turn allowed my mom a break. One of those first stays included Joey coming along with me. This was new for all four of us. Joey had never come along, and Bob and Diane never had two kids stay over before. They were amazed at how well "behaved" Joey was compared to me. I found this funny because I knew he was simply being polite, and I knew they weren't seeing the Dennis the Menace side of his personality, which we both shared. They would see some of his other side later that summer. And I'd have my chance to say "I told you so." I'm simply saying we're the same. He was no more well behaved than I was. We were "boys who would be boys."

As the months started winding down to summer, things started heating up in more ways than one. My mom and Kirk began to once again have problems in their relationship. While he continued to work in Galesburg, he was staying out for extended periods and eventually not coming home at all. This got my mom frustrated, and Elric, Elizabeth, and I were dragged along for it. At this point in the season, I was staying home from school on the hottest days because it was simply too hot to be stuck in a sweltering school bus for over fifty miles twice a day. There were a few days prior to that when I was suffering without relief during that bus ride. It was an oven, and it lasted for over two and a half hours. It's a torturous hellish experience when you can't sweat. But going with Mom meant tolerating the high temps in the van with no AC. Thus, it was no better than suffering on the school bus. The early peak of the situation happened on the day my mom confronted Kirk while he was at his new girlfriend's house. My brother Elric and I watched as my mom proceeded to punch out the window on the front door of Kirk's girlfriend. This got my mom sent to the ER, followed by a free trip to jail. This was actually the only time I ever saw my mom arrested. So now Kirk, who had somewhat responsibility for us, took Elric and me back home. He got us McDonald's for lunch, and my aunt Leslie ended up bailing my mom out of jail. This was just the early peak of a long summer, which would pretty much finally end their relationship. Due to previous experience, I did not nor did I want to go along for the ride.

Before or just as all the drama between Kirk and my mom began, Joey and I had our court date in Galesburg for the accident at McCabe Scrap Iron. Mom, Kirk, Joey, and I were all headed there, expecting a win-or-lose decision that very day. I remember being surprised when an attorney representing McCabe told me, "Good luck." He knew my grandmother somehow and was sympathetic toward what happened. After reviewing everything, the presiding judge announced he would make a decision within a few weeks. If he ruled in our favor, we would have enough money to buy a house and still have funds for my medical needs. My theory was Kirk left after I moved in for any or perhaps all of the following reasons—we weren't going to win the lawsuit, he couldn't handle my needs, or once again he was bored of my mom and wanted a new start with a new girlfriend. Kirk eventually would have taken off again anyway; that's just the way he was. Either way, I'm sure that us not winning the lawsuit against McCabe hastened his decision to leave and helped seal the end of his relationship with my mom. But my mom continued to struggle with accepting that fact for many months afterward.

Within a few days after the window-punching incident, my mom had been discussing with Diane and Bob for me to stay with them for a short time while my mom juggled trying to patch her relationship up with Kirk and preparing to move to a new place. I was still stuck at home because it was too hot to travel back and forth for school. So I stayed with the Wells for a few weeks. Early on, rules were set that we wouldn't go out for dinner and shopping every day. It wasn't a vacation or leisure stay. They had to work, and of course, I understood. A few times, I went with Diane to work, and I'd just chill in an empty room all day watching TV until we headed back home. I didn't mind going along, except for the fact that I was immobile and we both had to get up very early. Her trip to work was almost as long as mine to school, yet she woke up a little earlier than I usually did, because she had to get us *both* ready to go for the day. I couldn't tag along with Bob because, at the time, he worked as a mechanic in a garage with no air conditioning. That would not work at all, so Diane set it up with her nephew Donnie to hang out with me at home during the day. I had met him before, and he was a huge Disney fan, even more so than I was of anything at that time. I did like Disney afternoon cartoons and obviously toys, so it gave us something in common to talk about. He was actually the first person to point out to me that characters from different cartoons are often voiced by the same people. He told me the voice of Darkwing Duck was the same guy who voiced Don Karnage, Winnie the Pooh, and Tigger. I now know his name is Jim Cummings and he's done countless characters during his career, including Taz the Tasmanian Devil, as well as characters from video games I've played such as Star Wars: The Old Republic. That's part of why I love voice actors so much. One voice connects so many favorite characters and memories. Initially, when I went down to stay with Bob and Diane, I don't think I realized how long I was actually going to be there while the turmoil still went on back at home with my mom. Before I knew it, I actually missed the final day of school that year because it was still too hot to travel. Now summer break had arrived, and I was free from school obligations.

Chapter 13

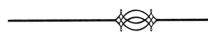

When June arrived, I once again had to go back to Galveston for evaluation. This time was different because Bob was flying with me, and it would be the first time in the new hospital since it was completed earlier that year. Either way, I was very apprehensive going down there again. I fully expected to be admitted and feared another summer of seemingly endless surgeries, procedures, loneliness, and pain. As usual, when I arrived, I was given a shower despite my objections and then sat in my room, watching TV. I didn't have my power chair that time because I couldn't bring it to Bob and Diane's place; thus, it was left at home. No power chair meant I was immobile, which made it all that much worse. The first evening, I went to bed, praying to God for a short stay so I could spend summer at home with my family instead of being stuck in a hospital, enduring painful surgeries one after another. I think it was the next day or two that I got good news from my therapist Merilyn my prayers to God had been answered. I remember telling her, "I actually don't think I need any surgeries right now." She then explained to me the doctors were holding off any surgeries for the time being and I would stay for a month of physical therapy. This worked for me, and I was glad I wouldn't be stuck there all summer. Therapy could be painful, but not as painful as it used to be, and I preferred it over surgery any day. Bob went back home as soon as we found out how long I'd be staying, and once again, I was alone, but this time, it would be easier.

Apart from the fact that I was immobile during my first stay, I enjoyed the welcome change of the new hospital. With eight floors, it was modernized, had spacious private rooms, and yes, it even had functioning AC with separate climate controls in each room. For me, the AC was a big plus. It meant no more fans and sweltering in the Texas heat. The new facilities on each floor were much larger than the old building too. The therapy area occupied the entire east end of the fourth floor, as well as the playroom taking up the entire west end of the third floor. The cafeteria was located on the west end of the roof and had outdoor areas on each corner. One of the coolest aspects of the building was the enclosed outdoor areas located throughout the building. They were brick and concrete rooms enclosed with steel bars on the outside and windows on the inside. This allowed patients to enjoy some outdoor air without actually leaving the hospital. The thunderstorm lover in me always thought it would be cool to watch a hurricane in one of them. For easy access, there were six elevators, three for patient and visitor use and three for staff and surgical use. On the second floor was a walkway connecting to the hospitals across the street. This made it easier to access needed facilities, such as X-rays, scans, and hearing aids, which the Shriners building didn't have without being forced to cross traffic on the streets or face the weather outside. There were even family accommodations in the building, which allowed family and/or patients to stay on-site without leaving, though I never needed to use them. Overall, I was very impressed and satisfied with the new building, and it greatly eased my stress and discomfort I had at the old building.

My first stay at the new hospital went smoothly for the most part. Physical therapy occupied a huge chunk of my day. It was simply a bit of stretching my limbs and skin in places that had stiffened over the past months since my time out of a hospital and daily therapy. Prior to that visit, I had been curious about asking for prosthetic ears. Initially, I wanted them because I wanted to get an earring, and I honestly didn't think I would be taken seriously, but they figured a prosthetic ear meant it would be easier for me to use a hearing aid. First, a plaster mold was made of the surface of what remained of my ear, and from there, the orthotics tech Roland Morales constructed the actual prosthetic. When it was done, all that required to attach it was a small brush of skin-friendly glue, and it was simply pressed into place. At the end of the day, it is simply taken it off, and the excess glue is wiped off with glue remover. It wasn't perfect though, because there was actually very little for the prosthetic to cling to. They would fall off quite often and thus had to be reattached. I didn't stop using them altogether until many years later.

Three times during my stay that month, I went out on day trips to enjoy some time outside of the hospital and see more of Galveston. Catherine took me out for ice cream and a visit to Moody Gardens. Back then, Moody Gardens was much smaller, and most of it was just a small beachfront water park. It was nice being out, and it was a cool place to see, but once again, it was a situation where I wish I wasn't stuck in a wheelchair. I wanted so badly to be able to get out of that chair and play in the flowing waterfall like the kids I saw as they splashed about. Not to mention the heat was starting to get to me and we decided to leave. We stopped at Taco Bell on the way back, but my body has a way of telling me when I've gotten too hot. Even when I'm already hungry, if I'm hot enough, I can't do anything until after I've thoroughly cooled off. When I'm that hot, it requires cool air and/or water-facilitated cooling along with simple rest. The limited movement allows my body to rest and my blood flow to redistribute the heat in my body so I cool down faster. And almost always, when I've gotten too hot, a headache usually follows, either during the overheating or just as I'm starting to cool off. Some joys in life had a price to pay, and overheating could be one of them.

A leisure trip or time out might be fun, but overheating would be a consequence if it was hot enough. The other trip was with the same nurse and her husband who took me to the flight museum the previous summer. Only this time we went to the Galveston Railroad Museum. Even though I am somewhat a fan of planes now, trains were always an interest of mine. My grandpa worked most of his life for the railroad in Galesburg, and as I kid, I always expected to be doing something along the same lines when I grew up. It was a nice museum and had several exhibits throughout, including the largest tank car union railroad ever built. I only wish Galesburg had a railroad museum that could match Galveston's. The final outing before I headed back home was an evening out with Catherine again. I had waited weeks to see *Batman Returns,* and I finally got the chance. I had a great time that night, and I always enjoyed our one-on-one time back in those days. Moments like those helped make up for what I missed out on. It also strengthened the friendship I had with people like Catherine and the nurse who took the extra time and effort to make my day brighter.

Before I move on, I must point out that I have indeed waited too long to get this next "incident" on paper. I remember her face, and she should consider herself lucky I don't remember her name and the fact that I never reported any of her crap to anyone. I simply couldn't, because I was alone, and I wasn't confident that whatever I might say wouldn't have repercussions back on me if I had then chosen to say something. She was the same nurse who had given me grief a few times during my stay the previous summer. Yes, the very same one who disturbingly dared me to stick my arm down her bra and reach for a $100 bill. The newest incident happened like a bolt out of the blue without warning or provocation. That's why I never forgot it, simply because I had done literally nothing to deserve it. Anyway, the nurses had just finished my daily care, and I was dressed and sitting in my wheelchair. After the other nurses had left the room, she remained behind, and suddenly, she had her face just inches from mine and abruptly blurted out, "Get out of my life." She then walked right out the door as I sat there dumbfounded, stunned, and taken aback as to what had just occurred. I was stuck there with nobody to talk to about what had just happened, and the thoughts flowed through my mind of what I had done to merit such a hateful snide comment. I never did anything hateful to her or anyone down there. I didn't cuss, I didn't hit, I didn't whine, I never talked back, and as I grew older, the only time I cried was in private or the rare occasions when my emotions got to me during a sad moment, such as simply being away from home. I was never around black people at home, and even before I was burned (though I had one bad experience with a black classmate when he punched me in the stomach), I had no prejudice at all toward them. As a burn survivor, I could sometimes face similar discriminations and hate, and I could at least begin to understand the racial tension some felt. So why did she harbor such ill will toward me? She wasn't that way with other patients, so why was I any different? I'll say it one last time—she's fortunate I don't remember her name. Luckily for her, she was no longer at Shriners when I returned for my next hospital stay months later, which made future stays that much easier.

My flight back home to Illinois before the Fourth of July holiday that year was simply the opposite of going to Galveston in the first place. Only the trip back didn't include the nervousness and apprehension of an impending hospital stay. When I returned, my mom had finished moving and was temporarily staying at the YMCA apartments in Monmouth. But in the meantime, I was still staying with Bob and Diane until Mom found a bigger and longer-term residence. I hadn't seen my mom and my siblings in over a month when they came to Canton and visited me on the 4th. At the time, the animated version of *101 Dalmatians* was somewhat popular, and Mom brought a poster for me. Amusingly, for me at least, Bob and

Diane saw Joey as just like me. While he was there, he was in and out of the door without closing it. I told you he wasn't more behaved than I was. When he stayed prior to that, he was simply on his best behavior. I'm not hinting anything; I'm just pointing out that Joey and I weren't much different, yet they still loved me all the same. That Fourth of July was my first outside the hospital. Even though I had been allowed a few hours with Catherine the year before, this time I didn't have to return to the hospital afterward. Bob, Diane, her brother Alan and his wife, and I all went out that evening and watched the fireworks from the bed of Bob's truck. There was an embarrassing moment for Alan that night, but I'm going to leave out the details. Let's just say I was being a smartass that night and announced Alan's dirty deed to everyone nearby. I was just joking around like I always do, and I never let Alan live it down after that; it's just more fun that way.

As the summer progressed, it wasn't long after the holiday when Mom finally moved into an apartment and I was home with my mom and siblings again. The Lincoln Homes apartment complex was a public housing project for low-income families. It was our first time living in an apartment, and with five kids in such a small space, my mom had her hands full. But it was the best she could do at the time. Western Illinois home health still came by every morn-ing and evening for daily bath care and therapy. Other than that, it wasn't much different than before, except for the fact that the apart-ment was much smaller than anywhere else we had been, and my mom was still trying to hold on to Kirk. The neighborhood itself was pretty nice for a few short weeks after I arrived. The kids in the neighborhood seemed to accept me. The first day back, as my mom and my brother introduced me to the neighborhood kids, one of them pushed my wheelchair around to the back of the apartment, pointed to a chair, and said, "What is this?" I said, "What the heck do you think it is? It's a chair." Just then, my mom came around the corner of the building and explained to the girl who asked the question that I was actually smarter than Joey. Seriously, folks, being burned doesn't affect the mind, only the body. Physically, my body and appearance may have been scarred and damaged, but other than the hidden and not so apparent emotional scars that any trauma survivor goes through, mentally I'm just the same as any other person. So I deserve the same respect and dignity as anyone else might be given. Whenever it happens, I do my best to ignore it, but I do tend to get annoyed when people ask me dumb questions or talk to me in a condescending or childish way. Try to look past my appearance and talk to me like you would anyone else.

A week or three after I had been at home, I was already going back to Diane and Bob's for a weekend stay. I was going to extend my stay, but I told them I missed the neighborhood kids and wanted to head home a little early. They drove me back up to Monmouth, but unfortunately, nobody was home, and we drove around all over, trying to find them. Bob and Diane were getting angry, and I felt somewhat guilty for asking them to bring me back early only for it to be a wasted trip. I never did find out where my mom and siblings had gone that day, but I assumed it possibly involved Kirk, as that seemed to be a reliable pattern at the time. Over the weeks, things quickly changed with the kids in the neighborhood. For whatever reasons, a few of the parents who were somewhat friendly with my mom and whose kids were friendly to us seemed to turn on us, partly because my mom was instable sometimes and vented a few of her frustrations publicly. But that was no reason for my siblings and me to be caught in the crossfire. Some of the kids seemed to flip back and forth from friendly to hostile. To be honest, I think their parents were under pressure from others to stop being friends with my mom altogether. From who, I don't know, but I do think Kirk's sister might have been part of it. I'll explain more on that later. But some of these kids showed such hate, and that hate trickled down to the youngest directly from the parents and older siblings, yet another example of me not understanding what I had done to deserve such rudeness. There was one little black girl in the neighborhood around two or three years old, and every time I saw her looking at me, she was making faces or even flipping me off. Adding insult to injury, her parents noticed what she was doing and didn't lift a finger. I'm hardly trying to paint the picture with myself as the innocent victim, but I just can't understand how any parent would let a small child behave that way toward anyone, especially when that person has a disability. Whatever happened to love thy neighbor and common decency toward your fellow human?

There was also one incident with one of the neighborhood black kids who had been coming over to our apartment to play video games. Joey and I quickly became aware that the boy and his brother were obviously only coming over to play on our Super Nintendo. As soon as it was shut off, they were out the door without saying a word. So in a sense, they were video game moochers. They didn't care about being friends; they were fakes who only wanted to use our games. But one day, while getting ready to leave with mom in our van, Joey had just told one of them they couldn't come over anymore just to use our Nintendo. The boy picked up a stick and was chasing Joey around the van while Mom was busy putting me in. Mom all the while was oblivious to the whole thing while Joey kept yelling, "Mommmmmm!" When she finally noticed, Mom grabbed the stick and simply took it from him. He ran off, and as my mom was just about to get into the van, the drama intensified when the boy's mom showed up and began bitching at my mom, as if her boy had been beaten blue. By her behavior, she made it seem like her son chasing and attacking my brother was okay. My mom was calm at first and attempted to defuse it by trying to leave. But the woman then slammed the door on my mom's head, pinning it between the door and the frame. Sure my mom isn't perfect, but in that case, she totally did not deserve any of it. I was pissed. I was only twelve, but I let out a slew of profanities, yelling at her to stay away from my mom. Had I been physically able to, I might have sought enough retribution to get myself arrested. In the end, justice was served, and the woman was arrested instead.

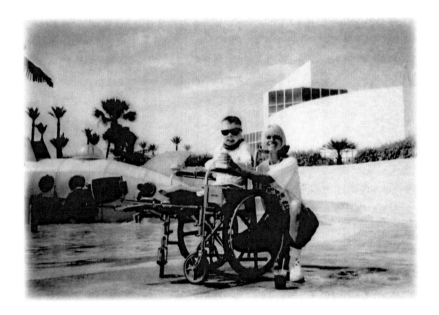

Chapter 14

When August came around, we started preparing for camp. Joey had gone the previous year, and his second time at camp would be my first. Monmouth and Galesburg firefighters pitched in on funds to help pay for a few things we still needed for camp. I think the most important of those was a sleeping bag for me. Just a few days before we left, a stray kitten came through the neighborhood and despite Mom's objections, my siblings and I didn't want to let it go. The kitten even got a mention in the newspaper article about Joey and me preparing for camp. But Mom still ended up taking the kitten to my aunt Lisa's, and like all pets we ever gave away, we never did see it again. Even though Joey, Mom, and the firefighters all told me I would have fun at camp, I was extremely hesitant to go. For weeks prior, I insisted to Mom I wasn't going and truly had no desire to. I know in my mind that my mom simply needed a break from dealing with both Joey and me, and it seemed, to me at least, like she was just trying to dump us on somebody else for a week. My reluctance to go was due to three reasons. The first was the fact I would obviously be around other kids. I had enough trouble dealing with neighborhood kids and staring from kids in public, and so I assumed I might have similar problems at camp. Second was simply my shyness when I was around new people. My hearing tended to make it hard to talk to people and make friends.

Also, my hearing goes along with the big main reason I didn't want to go, and that was my special needs. I didn't have just one or two needs; I had a whole bunch. Most things people can do for themselves every day were the things I needed help with—dressing, bathing, hygiene, wound care, eating, etc. And don't forget the physical therapy and any garments I was still wearing or the fact that I would be in my portable wheelchair, which meant being forced to rely on somebody else to push me around. I was still twelve years old, and I really didn't take much of an active role in how my care was done. Camp would be different, because my counselors would be new to the situation just like me. Just a day or two before we left, even Joey had concerns when I heard him say to Mom, "I'm not so sure about this." Even though he knew how much fun it was, he too was uncertain about me going to camp.

It seemed I had no choice; despite all my concerns and objections, I was going to camp whether I wanted to or not. We got up very early that Sunday morning, around 5:00 a.m. Keith Patterson at the time was a firefighter from Monmouth, and he picked us up that morning. I had already met him prior, and as we said goodbye to Mom and left, I thought to myself that with just Joey and Keith, everything was okay so far, but that didn't last long at all. From Monmouth, we went to Galesburg Fire Department, where we transferred to another van with Galesburg firefighters and another first time camper named Jimmy Palmer. From there, it was a quiet ride to Moline, where we picked up another camper. Our ride to camp was a long five to six hours. That first year, we avoided the interstate and toll ways for the majority of the trip. This was especially true when we got closer to the suburbs. On the way up, we stopped to eat breakfast at Hardee's, and that was the first example of my anxiety about camp. I didn't have my eating tool, which meant I couldn't feed myself. So to my embarrassment, I explained I couldn't feed myself, and one of the adults with us helped me out. When we arrived at camp, everything was still quiet. That first year at camp, we arrived before any other campers. Whether this was intentional or not, I never found out, but it did help me slowly ease in and become more comfortable without the unwanted stress from being around other kids and just suddenly overwhelmed by sensory overload because of too much going on at once. I admit I assumed it would stay that quiet and calm, but it wasn't meant to be. And to be totally honest, I'm grateful it wasn't. But like I said, a calm transition into camp was easier than a chaotic one. The hardest part about that day, believe it or not, was the simple act of the first time when I told my counselor Mike I had to pee.

A typical day at camp during those early years started with flag up around 8:00 a.m. All the cabin groups would then meet at the lodge for flag-up and the pledge of allegiance. Then we did morning exercise until the dinner bell was rang, letting everyone know our meal was ready. We then went inside to our cabin tables, and when all was quiet, we all sang our praise to the Lord, thanking him for our food. The first few years at camp, aside from morning prayer, there were two rituals during mealtime. The first was that whenever you were seen with your elbows on the table, eventually somebody would shout your name, and a song followed about how rude it was to put your elbows on the table. But it didn't end there. After the song, you were expected to get up from your seat, run out either end of the lodge, and come back through the other end. Sometimes, the accused was even made to run back the other way. The other song was just for fun. An individual or sometimes entire cabin group would be asked to show us "how they get down." So they either ignored it and were booed or stood up at the table and did a little dance. Both those rituals kept mealtimes quite loud until it stopped years later. I assume the loudness and the longer mealtimes we had are the reason it eventually ended. Oh well, it meant more time for other things after meals. For me, back then, I usually had my shower and morning care just after breakfast. Mike Kilburg said about my showering, "We had to figure out how to bathe you without either drowning you or dropping you and not making it too uncomfortable." So as I mentioned before, I was new to camp, but so were my counselors. We were all learning as we went along. Also, at the time, my care still included daily physical therapy to limit my skin tightening and stiffening so that was remedied by therapy at the Health Center. For fun, our afternoon activities consisted of choosing something to do during "skill periods." That included crafts, fishing, team's course, life journals, etc. Many of the activities at the start of the week focused on team building. On the first day, the most effective and fun was the team's course. The entire cabin would have to work together to solve a problem/puzzle presented to us. They all involved some kind of physical challenge, and it focused on teaching teamwork and trust in your team to accomplish a common goal. I still remember the trust exercise in my first year. The exercise involved standing on a raised platform and falling flat backward onto the crossed arms of the cabin groups. The person falling had to let himself fall naturally and trust that the group will catch them. Jim Allen was so afraid of the height he was in tears, but in the end, we convinced him to trust us, and he fell safely, and by the end of team's course, our social walls were coming down, and already, we were more cohesive and becoming comfortable with each other. Then typically there was usually an all-camp nightly activity for everyone to enjoy. The first few years, we had a number of different nightly activities throughout the week. The usual activities included capture the flag, muckman suitcase, puppet show, and others I can't remember. But the one we never missed has always been the yearly dance. That in a rather small nutshell sums up what camp was like. To be honest, I can go on and on with every little detail, and the activities varied from year to year, and things change, but I always enjoyed myself and the people I spent my time with while I was there. The most difficult aspect of that first year obviously was my physical care and needs. Like I said, my counselors were rookies, and they had to learn about my needs as we went along. Getting showered, wound care, and daily dry-skin treatment back then was a learning process, and back then, my needs were greater than they are now. Then there were those times when I overheated. The first few years of camp were held in mid-August, when the temperatures were still too hot for my comfort most of the time. Just about every year, at least once I would overheat enough to require facilitated cooling. Back then and even today actually, the most effective way was with cold water, and on more than one occasion, I was literally hosed down with a garden hose to cool my body off. To this day, I'm still used as an example during camp orientation training about full thickness burns, the inability to sweat, and the resulted overheating.

That first year at camp was an unforgettable experience that changed my life forever. Like Christmas or other special holidays, camp would eventually be a part of my life I couldn't imagine living without. At camp, the stress, worries, and problems of being burned stayed at home and sometimes faded away altogether. Camp was the only place I felt I could truly connect with peers my own age. At home or other places, sometimes I could be friendly with kids younger than myself, but I lacked friendships with anyone closer to my own age. If I remember correctly, my counselors that first year were Mike Herbert, Mike Kilburg, Scott Vaughn, LJ Kielczynski, Phil Griffith, and Dave Poore, and we were staying in cabin Silver Maple. Mike Herbert, my cabin leader that year, was actually one of Joey's counselors from the year before. I'm somewhat shy and can seem like I want to be alone, but my counselors and the boys from my cabin brought me out of my shell, so to speak. Mike Kilburg was the first counselor from my cabin to approach me and introduce himself. When I asked him to write down some thoughts about our first year at camp and our friendship since then in his own words, he told me he knew about the extent of my burns and wondered just what the hell he got himself into. Needless to say, he was nervous, but then again, we all were. When the van pulled up and he saw me, he thought to himself, *There is no time like the present,* as he came over to introduce himself saying, "Caper, my name is Mike, and no matter what, we are going to have fun this week." I had my special needs, but everyone in that cabin helped make me feel like I was truly one of the guys, not a disabled boy who could only be handled delicately with kid gloves. That first year, I think the most fun were the times when our cabin group was doing something together. Whether it was mealtime, afternoon activities, hanging out in our cabin, or the all-camp nightly activity, we were bonded. Not all that different from soldiers at war who become brothers. We may not have witnessed the hardships of war, but we bear scars and memories that give us a brotherly bond. As the week progressed, the visible scars were no longer relevant to us. We shared a common bond through our experiences as burn survivors, and thus, we were stronger because of it. A burn survivor faces many challenges in life that come and go endlessly. Those challenges can make life difficult, and for some, it makes them feel like they have nobody to turn to or connect with, as if nobody understands the adversities we go through on a daily basis. Just looking in the mirror, we are reminded every day by our scars that those hardships are never ending, but they can be easier with the support from people who *do* understand and do care. Burn camp was the first place outside a hospital where I felt the support and connection from others who do understand what I've been through and vice versa. The support goes both ways, and I do believe the healing never ends. I may be scarred, and because of those scars, I appear and seem different than others, but I promise you, I'm not broken. I persevere despite the hardships, and I'm forever thankful for all the friendships I've made at camp over the years, and I constantly do my best to return the favor.

I became close with all the counselors in my cabin that year, but for me, I had the strongest friendships with Mike Kilburg and Scott. During writing this book, I have asked a few people if they could contribute toward the overall story, so those who read it could see the perspective from people I've met and formed friendships with. I always asked for something simple, and some ended up writing a little more than others. The following few paragraphs is Scott Vaughn's account about that special first year at camp. It's the longest contribution from anyone in this book, but in his exact words, he wrote, "I hope it's not too long, but asking me to put my first year with you in a single paragraph is like asking someone to paint a landscape on the head of a pin." That indeed is true because even I find it hard to convey the important aspects of that year at camp, let alone everything that I could possibly put into words. Anyway, here is what Scott had to say about our first year. "The first-year burn camp was held at Camp Duncan in 1991, I went on visitors' day to see what it was all about. What I saw immediately made me want to come back the next year as a counselor. I saw campers playing everywhere, doing all kinds of activities. Kids were swimming, boating, and fishing on the lake. At the front of the lodge was a line of campers and staff waiting to play foursquare. They even had an archery range. I knew that all these kids were burn survivors, and to see them running and laughing seemingly without a care in the world made me so happy for them. Collectively, I could see the bond that had formed between the campers and the staff, most of whom I had never even met before the start of camp, just a few days earlier. This, I thought, was something I wanted to be a part of.

"At the time, my three children were all still very young, so as a father, I hadn't yet gotten to experience this type of activity with my own kids. So the next year when I was accepted as a volunteer counselor for burn camp 1992, I couldn't wait to take part in all the classic summer camp activities with the campers.

"A few weeks before the start of camp, I got a call from one of the camp directors. She said, 'We don't normally do this, but I wanted to give you some advanced information on your camper.'

"Camper? As in one? I knew the counselors at burn camp were assigned in teams to a group of campers, not just one. This was odd. She went on to describe Caper and his injuries. 'He lost both his arms and both his legs.' My first thought was, *Camp isn't going to be anything like what I thought it would be.*

"She went on to tell me that I and one other firefighter were being assigned as Caper's counselors for the week. Fortunately for me, that other firefighter was Mike Kilburg. Mike's energy was endless, his personality was infectious, and his sense of humor was one of a kind.

"The counselors arrived at camp a few days before the campers to learn the rules and expectations and mostly to work on team building. I had a great time meeting and working with some amazing people, but I was also nervous about meeting Caper. The thought of his injuries didn't bother me, but what did was the thought of not living up to the responsibilities that had been placed on Mike and me. Burn camp was a place where young burn survivors could come to play, interact, and be a kid without the insensitive stares and comments they were subject to in their everyday lives. Caper deserved those freedoms as much as any other kid there. How were we going to make camp fun for him? Answer: we didn't. He did.

"As soon as the kids arrived at camp, our week with Caper quickly took on a life of its own. The first thing I noticed was his interaction with the other campers. For the first time since he was burned, or so I assumed, young children were running to him rather than away. Their scars hadn't affected their natural curiosity as children, and being burn survivors themselves, they knew it was okay to ask what had happened. Because his injuries were so severe, I got the feeling that being around Caper gave some of them a sense of feeling normal that they hadn't felt since they got burned. I'm sure he didn't realize it at the time, but Caper had become an instant role model.

"Once the parents and escorts left and the regular camp activities got rolling, it became clear that my week wasn't going to consist of sitting under a tree, trying to make idle conversation with a handicapped twelve-year-old kid. Every time we asked Caper if he wanted to try something, the answer was yes. It was as if his spirit was completely unaware of the injuries his body had suffered. During the next week, Caper went fishing on the lake, drove the boat, went swimming in the pool, participated in arts and crafts, and even shot arrows on the archery range. One of my favorite moments was during visitors' day when a group of firefighters who were specialists in rope rescue rigged up a zip line and special harness for Caper's wheelchair and sent him zip-lining down the hill next to the lodge.

"I don't know about Mike, but about halfway through the week, I started looking forward Caper's daily physical therapy sessions with the angels in the health center since it meant a little downtime for us. Between his special needs and his desire to take advantage of everything camp had to offer, being Caper's counselor was pretty exhausting. And if the physical toll wasn't enough, there was the emotional element that was always there. Even though it was only for a week, spending twenty-four hours a day with someone who'd been injured that badly, especially a kid, was tough for me. On one especially hot day when we stayed inside to escape the heat, I remember watching Caper reading a book and was amazed at how proficient he was at turning the pages with his hooks. But my fascination was offset by sadness as I thought how no child should be that good at using prosthetic hands.

"But if I had to describe the overall experience of my first year at burn camp in one word, that word would be *awestruck*. I was awestruck by the camaraderie of the volunteer staff and counselors who were mostly strangers when they were thrown head-first into this swarm of boundless adolescent energy.

"I was awestruck by the environment that the IFSA camp committee had created. Our mission was simple and clear: 'To provide a safe environment for children who have experienced significant burn injuries in a nonjudgmental atmosphere in which children have the opportunity to build their self-esteem as they enjoy the varied activities that make up their camp experience.' We were never allowed to forget that everything we said and did was for the purpose of successfully meeting that mission. I was awestruck by the strength and resolve of the campers. And mostly, I was awestruck by this kid named Capernicus and how he overcame what should have killed him. Since we became friends, I've learned to appreciate a lot more things that I used to take for granted. He continues to be one of my most positive role models to this day."

As the week went on, I felt completely at ease, as if I had found a new home. During the course of the week, I formed more friendships and lifelong bonds than I can even remember. But I think it was just the day before we headed home that Kim Kiser, who is the executive director at Camp Duncan, asked if I would like to see her cockatiels she was raising. I think I remember telling her earlier on in the week how much I liked birds and how I had always wanted one. For years, I actually wanted to be an ornithologist, so you can imagine my surprise and joy when she asked me if I wanted one. I was so excited and amazed somebody I had only known a few days would be generous enough to give me something like that, which I had wanted for so long. Kim asked which one I would like, and I said, "The one with the wolf whistle." Then she asked if I had a name for it, and I thought Duncan would be a great name. It would be a great reminder of the special place where I got him. Friday was typically a day of cabin awards and graduations. In those days, we would have the ceremony down on the outdoor chapel built into the hillside. Each cabin would be called up one by one as campers from each cabin were given personalized awards, like most quiet, best dancer, and loudest snorer. Then staff awards depending on how long you've been coming to camp, but those were few, considering it was the second year, and then finally ending with the graduation of the sixteen-year-old campers because that was the age limit. Throughout the ceremony, everyone was allowed to say something about their week, and counselors talked about how great their cabin group was. Friday night marked the best night activity, the all-camp dance. Keith "Doc" Patterson came all the way from Monmouth just to DJ for us. Doc was great at what he does and was always a highlight of the week. He knew I liked Bon Jovi, and over the years, he never failed to play at least one song dedicated to me and made sure I was up front and center every time.

The worst part about camp, you ask? Leaving. As the week went by in a blur, everyone began to realize that it's almost over until next year. The last two days are a tsunami of emotions, as campers and counselors reflect on their week at camp and say their good-byes to new friends and old. At the end of every day at camp, before all cabin groups head to bed, we have our friendship circle. Our final circle is just before the campers begin boarding their buses and arranged transportation to head home. A few words are said about the day or, in the final day, a few comments about the week. Then only after everyone is holding hands in one large circle, we begin to sing.

Friends I will remember you
Think of you
And pray for you
And when another day is through
I'll still be friends with you

And it's repeated once more. I always smile to myself when new counselors and anyone outside our camp family hears us sing the song. It's new and fresh to them, but it's almost as if they can see the harmony of our friendships reflected in our song. Then we all get on our buses, vans, etc., and our counselors seem to take forever saying good-bye. But Joey and I never say good-bye. Ironically, it's one of my favorite Bon Jovi songs, but it's a motto we both live by, "Never say good-bye." Good-bye is forever, so we always say, "See you later." Everywhere you look, you can see either a camper or counselor crying and saying, "See you next year." It seems like we never leave and everyone is always trying to stretch out every last second and won't let go, but inevitably, the time comes when we depart. We look out the van windows and can see people crying as we drive off. For Joey and the other boys and me, we are still half-wired up about our week, but as we head home, we grew quiet as our long ride went on. When we got home, I told Mom about camp and how awesome it was. I mentioned the dinnertime songs, my friends, counselors, the crafts I made, and of course, my new cockatiel from Kim. For the most part, I was fine until sometime later I just suddenly seemed to crash. The entire week, it seemed most of us were on an adrenaline high, and suddenly, it hit me like a ton of bricks how much I missed camp. I think I might have been listening to music, which for me can be a stress-relieving trigger, but nevertheless, I was crying, and my mom came into the living room and asked what was wrong. I'm comfortable enough with my emotions to admit saying, "I miss camp, Mom." After that, it's a half blur as I release the emotions. And to be totally honest, that wasn't the only year it happened, but after that, I did most of my emotional release, and post-camp wind down in private, my own way.

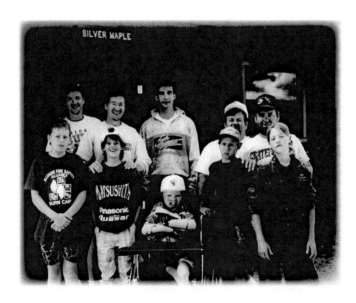

Chapter 15

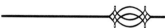

Camp was still very much on my mind for weeks after we got back home. It was evident in the nightly dreams about camp that it had made a lasting impression on me. But less than a week after camp ended, it was time once again for the dreaded back-to-school routine and the start of my seventh-grade school year. Because of the heat, I missed a few days at the start, but when I finally returned, a few of my classmates asked about where I had been. For the most part, the start of the school year was uneventful as the season progressed into the fall and my thirteenth birthday on October 4. My mom bought a *101 Dalmatians* cake, and a few neighbor kids were allowed to enjoy some also. It wasn't a huge bash or anything, and I didn't receive much, but in hindsight, it was better than nothing at all, though most of the kids there simply wanted free cake. My mom gave me audiotape cassettes for recording music on my stereo. That is just about the same time when my mom and I began having arguments. For example, one of those arguments was about how I felt as if Mom buying new bikes for all three of my younger siblings overshadowed my birthday. But feeling left out and jealous about material things wasn't the only issue. Increasingly, I was getting frustrated with the fact that my siblings were getting away with just about everything with hardly any punishment. For example, one day I approached

Elric and a neighborhood boy his age cutting up an old recliner chair with a kitchen knife in a field across from our apartment complex. As I got closer, Elric said, "Get out of here, or I'll cut you." You can imagine my anger when he said that. If I had been able to, I would have beaten him silly just for uttering those words, let alone threatening me. Victor would have done the same to me if I had been dumb enough to say something like that when I was younger. I told Mom immediately, and what did she do about it? Nothing at all. Tensions were increasing for multiple reasons. Mom was trying to raise five kids aged one to thirteen by herself. Kirk wasn't written off yet, but by then he pretty much wasn't playing any part in helping either. He definitely was no longer present, and I'm not sure whether he was still helping financially or not. Mom was still trying to hold on to him and get him back, but so far, it had been to no avail. Eventually, I remember one night our tensions came to a boil with Mom and me arguing after Joey accidently hit my wheelchair's joystick and rammed me into the stove, seriously bumping my leg and hurting it like hell. As Mom and I argued the words finally came out of my mouth, "You know I'm about ready to leave just like Victor did." If I didn't have my special needs, had been lesser burned or no burns at all but still in that living situation, I possibly might have ended up moving in with my grandparents if they would have allowed it, but I didn't have that option.

I don't remember exactly when, but one day that fall upon returning home from school around four or so in the afternoon, a few familiar faces were waiting. Tyke Jordan, who was the fire chief from Galesburg Fire Department and a counselor from camp, Keith Patterson, and a few others donated a brand-new manual wheelchair to me. The one I had at the time wasn't very compact, which made it more difficult to fold and lift into a vehicle. The newer one was better suited to my needs because it would be many years until I had a van with a wheelchair lift enabling me to take my power wheelchair.

Bob and Diane came and picked me up for a weekend shopping trip once or twice that fall. They had even stopped by during my time at camp only to find me gone. I still remember the birthday present they gave me—*The Simpsons: Bart's Nightmare* for Super Nintendo. On top of that, they still took me out to lunch and shopping that day even though they had already given me the game. I looked forward to Halloween that year despite all the turmoil going on with everything. But for the most part, it was a huge disappointment. It was raining, and when we did try to go out even though other trick-or-treaters were also out and about, nobody seemed to give me or my siblings candy. Not even Kirk's sister Theresa and aunt of my youngest three sibs give us any. She said she didn't have any, but I swear she gave some to the next group who rang her doorbell. I could be wrong, but who knows. I had made up my mind—it was finally official for me that neighborhood sucked "donkey." Mom at least tried entertaining us by letting us bob for apples. But because of my jaw and lips, I found it pretty much impossible for me, and of course, I would rather have been out filling up my bag with free candy like I used to with my older cousin Chad in Farmington for Halloween '88 and '89. He always asked for a handful when we were done, but it was worth it because we stayed out until folks refused to hand us any-more. I think it was very early November when I was scheduled to go back to Galveston for a checkup and possibly more reconstructive surgeries. My mom had given me ten bucks for whatever while I was down there, but she had to stay home, and once again, I was going to fly down with Bob. When the time came for whatever reason, I don't recall the details, but there was a communication problem with everyone involved, and I ended up not going. Obviously, it didn't bother me, because I was almost certain I would be facing another surgery. I'd much rather put up with family squabbles then be down in Galveston facing another round of surgeries.

Thanksgiving that year wasn't anything special. We stayed home, and we actually didn't have much for our "turkey day." Mom cooked a frozen turkey loaf, which actually tasted pretty good, but it wasn't much after it was split between all of us. Almost every night, I was still having dreams of being back at camp again, so you can imagine how excited I was when I arrived home from school one day to see my counselors Mike Kilburg, Mike Herbert, and Scott Vaughn waiting for me. They were there to take Joey and me to Chicago for the weekend. When we were being driven up to camp that year, we asked if we would be going through Chicago, but we were told we were going around it. I had actually wanted to see it because neither of us had been to a large city other than Denver, Colorado, back in 1988 or the outer parts of Houston, Texas, whenever we flew in and out of the airport for visits to the hospital in Galveston. The entire drive up there, we we're excited as we talked about what we would be doing that weekend. As we got closer, I said to Joey, "Wow, look, there are four lanes." One of the guys laughed at that simple comment, but you see things differently when you're younger. In my opinion, a child's perspective is one of the things that make childhood so great. Our first night we stayed at Mike Herbert's apartment and ordered out for pizza. We were doing stuff we never got to do when we were younger—just hanging out with positive male figures who genuinely wanted to be there for us. We had uncles and guy cousins, but none really spent time and mentored us like those guys did. So it's easy to understand why Joey and I consider them all our extended family and "brothers." That first night is still easy to remember. I lay awake on the couch, trying my best to get to sleep, but my attempt at falling asleep was pointless. I was simply too excited to sleep, and I soon realized Joey was also "sleepless in Chicago." He helped me sit up on the couch and gave me a drink of water. We were both excited about the next day, and we talked about the things we might see and do. After a few minutes, our restless young minds finally decided to hop off the highway and hit a rest area so we could get to sleep. The next day was Saturday, and pretty much everything they had planned for us was crammed into that one day. It might seem like a lot now, but back then, we had the energy for it. Our first stop was Brookfield Zoo. I had been to smaller zoos before, but Brookfield was way bigger than those. I saw the same primate house where a three-year-old boy fell into a gorilla enclosure in 1996. But I must say the most fun part was actually the dolphin show, because it was something Joey and I had never gotten to see before. Also, keep in mind, back then I didn't have the luxury of a power wheelchair when traveling, so I had to rely on others for pushing me around the entire zoo. It's fine, but nothing compares with the independence of freely maneuvering and moving around on your own free will. Because it was November, the lively colors of spring and summer were not present, and in their place, everything was brown or withered, signaling change and the oncoming winter. Little did I know a big change would soon be coming in the days ahead.

Our next stop after Brookfield Zoo was downtown Chicago. We ate at McDonald's for lunch, and I had never seen so many people packed at a McDonald's in my life. Joey still dislikes intense high-capacity crowds such as conventions because of the stares and unwanted attention I get, but for a place where people eat, the number of folks there back then was a new experience altogether. Next, we went up to the top of John Hancock Tower for yet another new experience. Unexpectedly, even to me, it was one I wasn't comfortable with once we were actually up there. I enjoy flying, and I loved climbing trees and high places when I was younger, but for some reason, I was very nervous. The closer I got to those windows, the more intense my fear. No matter what I did, I couldn't shake it off. Part of me was curious and wanted to see what was out there, but my fear said, "No way, stay back." To be honest, I think part of that fear comes from the loss of control. I was being pushed around in a wheelchair with no control of movement, and whether it makes sense or not, it does make a difference. Years later, I went back with a power chair, and I was still nervous, but because I had more control than on the first visit, I was at least able to push that fear a step or two further, and I got closer to the window than the first time. After we left the tower, we then went across the street to FAO Schwarz, a three-story toy store we could only dream of. The place was amazing, but the pre-holiday crowds and the prices were just a bit too much. Then finally, from there, we headed to the northern suburbs, where we stayed the night with Scott Vaughn and his family. Scott was different from my other counselors, because at the time he was the only one with kids of his own. His two youngest boys, Brian and Corey, who were twins and a little shy, and their older sister Kelly, they all welcomed Joey and me as if we had known them for years. On Sunday after we left Scott's, we stopped by a very recognizable landmark—the famous house used for filming *Home Alone*. It was yet another new experience for Joey and me. I loved that movie and had never gotten to see in person something I had only seen on film. It gave the movie more depth and made it feel more real knowing it was a real place that I could see and *almost* touch. From there, we went back downtown to Madison stadium to see the famous Ringling Bros. and Barnum & Bailey Circus. So much was crammed into that weekend in Chicago I almost forgot about the circus, and I'm sure there are parts I don't remember. But on our way home, I do remember we actually had to call home when we were near the Quad Cities area because we were unsure which way to go. I'm a very good navigator, but that only applies to places I've previously been, plus the night made recognizing landmarks that more difficult, but we made it home okay in the end. It was an awesome weekend I got to share with Joey and the guys. Not only did Joey and I get to spend time together without our youngest three siblings, but it was the beginning of our friendships with our counselors outside of burn camp.

I remember a lot was going on at home and school during October and November. Somebody stopped by school one day to ask me a few questions about how things were going at home. The specific questions I remember were those like "Did your mom ever leave you unsupervised or alone?" I did say that sometimes I went out to a grassy field near our apartments to be alone sometimes, and I answered the questions honestly. As for going out in the field by myself, I didn't let being in a wheelchair stop me. If I wanted to be alone with my thoughts, I believed I had the right to do so. Diane had mentioned before that she didn't want to see me end up in foster care, but she knew it could happen. I, on the other hand, feared it, but I honestly didn't think it would happen. Mom told me one day about being angry with the school because she couldn't make it to my parent-teacher conference. She quoted something about kids, money, and distance. And to be honest, I agreed with her. It was almost fifty miles one way for an unemployed single mother of five, not an easy task. A few days after our Chicago trip was my school field trip to Wildlife Prairie Park, located just outside Peoria. When I was burned, I missed my fourth-grade field trip to the same place, and I had been there before in '89, but Mom decided to cut our visit short before we got to the actual animal habitat areas of the park. The park is accessible to wheelchairs for the most part. But in some places, even a power wheelchair needed assistance getting over larger bumps. I remember eating my lunch on a deck about forty to fifty feet above an open area with deer and elk. Everyone was scattered around eating lunch while I shared my Cheetos with the deer. My mom had given me five bucks for a souvenir, and being the bird lover that I was, I bought a small hand-carved cardinal, and my mom actually still has it. I think we both see it now as a memento of things before the next big change that was approaching.

Chapter 16

It was a school day late November, and it began no different than the rest of them, except for one small detail—my home health nurse that morning noticed a small bump similar to a blister on my chin. I honestly didn't think it was a big deal. I couldn't feel, see it, nor did it really affect me early on that day. But after I got to school that day, my teachers and aides quickly noticed that this so-called bump didn't look right. I thought the issue was being blown out of proportion and everyone was overreacting to a little bump. Diane showed up at the school and told me I was going to the hospital to have the bump looked at. I'm not fooled easily. My hearing may not be great, but I quickly notice body language when things aren't right. Diane wasn't the only one to show up that day. Questions and concerns were swirling all around, and I knew this had something to do with the questions I was asked by the DCFS (Department of Children and Family Services) worker previously. Of course, the new DCFS case-worker who showed up that day before I went to the hospital was an obvious tipoff. When I didn't go home on the bus that day, I started getting nervous. Diane took me to the hospital, and I was admitted back into the rehab floor I left months prior. Not only was I nervous about all the drama surrounding me, but the bump on my chin was bigger than I thought and still increasing in size. It was my first time dealing with a boil, but obviously, my concern was how much it was going to hurt. Diane explained it was just like a blister, that I wouldn't feel a thing, and that it just needs to be drained, so to speak. I was still nervous when the doctor came at my throat with a pair of small scissors. But it was my throat, why wouldn't I be? Thankfully, what Diane said was indeed true, and I felt no pain. It was simply a little poking and prodding to get the ugly bump to drain. I never did get another one on my neck after that. But over the years, I've had just a few in different places. The symptoms typically included the bump being sore to the touch and, in some cases, feeling ill just before it "pops" on its own, but when that happens, *ughhh*, the smell is terrible. Within a day or two in the hospital, my mom called and said, "Why didn't you say anything about your neck?" I was dumbfounded. How the heck was I supposed to know? I couldn't see it, I felt fine, and I was only thirteen. I never had one before, and it wasn't my job to know those things. That is the responsibility of parents and caretakers, not the child.

It was apparent to me I wasn't going home anytime soon. I met my new DCFS caseworker Mary while at school, and I think I remember her also stopping by the hospital. Diane and maybe Mary straight up explained to me I would be going to a foster home after my stay at Methodist. I tried to tell Diane how bad it would be thinking the only kind of foster home that would accept a kid with my needs must be some kind of residential facility, a cold child factory, which in my opinion wasn't much different than a hospital. I even said, "But they probably don't even have a Super Nintendo." Diane tried to assure me they probably did and explained she would be able to visit often. The foster home was in Rapatee, which was about seventeen miles from her house in Canton. This at least helped to ease my fears of moving in with people I've never met before. But before I could actually leave the hospital, I had to meet my new foster mom. As with any new face, I was nervous but even more so because I would soon be living with this person. I was in my room, watching TV, when Diane entered, and we were all introduced. Her name was Vicki Davis, and with her was her oldest foster daughter named Charlene. It's been a while, but I think she was about two to three years older than me. Anyway, the main reason for meeting me now instead of at her house or the day she picked me up was that Diane needed to teach her a few things about my needs. This would have been less stressful for me if Charlene hadn't accompanied Vicki. One stranger seeing me vulnerable is bad enough, let alone two and the second basically a sibling, so to speak. But at least she didn't bring along anyone else, I guess. Diane told her about my daily hygiene ritual, which was bathing followed by wound care and full-body dry-skin cream, which back then I used Eucerin cream, as well as dressing, eating, therapy, my more private needs, etc. Western Illinois Home Health would still be providing in home care, but Vicki would still need to know the basics and what I could not yet do for myself or needed help with.

Everyone involved continued to assure me that I had nothing to worry about, and Diane especially reminded me she would be close by if I needed her. Finally, the day came in very late November or early December when I was "shipped" to my new home. Okay, I wasn't actually shipped. Vicki came to the hospital that day, and Diane escorted us both out when I was leaving. I was still tense, but at least on the ride to Rapatee, it was just Vicki and I. On the ride there, she talked about the family and all the kids and even mentioned her brother's stepson Patrick, who was a classmate of mine in fourth grade back in Yates City. She asked me about my favorite foods, toys, etc. anything, which I know now she was getting me to let my guard down and just learn what I liked and enjoyed so she could try to make my transition easier. The closer we got to Rapatee, the more I was trying to figure out where it was. We went through Farmington and proceeded west past Middle Grove and the Midland

Coal Company. And then not much further at all was Rapatee. Oh, so this little town was Rapatee. No wonder I didn't remember where it was; the town was so small it had no post office and just a few occupied homes. I'd only been through it a handful of times, but Diane was right about it being close to Canton, and we drove through there every time I went to stay at her place prior to then. I never told anyone, but my earliest memory of Rapatee was actually when I was about five or so years old I was with my grandparents when we stopped at the antique store directly next to the house I would someday live in. How do I know it's the same place? Every time I went through Rapatee after that first time with my grandparents, I noticed the same things from that memory. The tables and lone tree in front of the shop, the no-gas gas station down the road, and even the high school down the road all fit into that memory. So I did remember the town, but it was so small it didn't linger in my mind.

Arrival at the house was the step I was dreaded. I would see what kind of place it was, and all those new eyes would be on me. It was too much attention for my comfort, and to make it worse, they were all kids except for Vicki's husband, Lee. Remember, kids in general made me nervous because I disliked the staring and attention and never knew how they might react around me. I'm shy enough as it is, and all the initial attention didn't help things. I honestly admit that I was greeted warmly and did feel welcome, so that was a good thing at least. In order from youngest to oldest were David Edwardson (aged eight), Mystic Harman (aged ten), Gregg Edwardson (aged ten), Kyle Harman (aged twelve), Jessica Haulk (aged fifteen), and Charlene Davis (aged sixteen). David and Gregg were obviously brothers. Kyle and Mystic were siblings and Vicki's own children. Jessica was on her own, like me, and Charlene had been adopted by Vicki and Lee. I must point out that I never called them Mom and Dad. It's not that they didn't fill the role, and it wasn't personal in any way. I just didn't believe in calling anyone but my own mom in that way. Diane and Bob also played those roles, but I never flat out said it. It was implied, but that's entirely different. I also must mention that Lee Davis was Vicki's third husband. It's nothing important, but with all the last names and different parents floating around, it can get confusing. I was destined to share a room with Kyle on the converted porch bedroom. I hated the idea of sharing a room at all, but I had little choice in the matter. That first evening, Diane stopped by, which eased my tension, and Dean, my home nurse, was there also. Unfortunately, because of the distance, Dean would not be my home nurse any longer, and new nurses would be taking over in place of those I had back in Monmouth. The first dinner we had was tacos because I had told Vicki how much I loved them. Keep in mind I was still adapting to feeding myself, and tacos were still pretty much impossible for me to feed myself at the time unfortunately. Prior to eating, Charlene asked me if she could feed me, and to avoid hurt feelings, I said yes. But when the food was ready, I simply said, "I changed my mind," and allowed Vicki to do so instead. After all, it was still my first night, and I would gradually ease into things at my own pace. The most awkward and embarrassing moment that night was when Kyle could see in full view everything going on when Dean and Diane were explaining and showing things to Vicki concerning my care. My body was my business, and unless you are a nurse or a parental-guardian figure, I didn't want anyone seeing the scars and vulnerability of me unclothed.

I settled in pretty fast at my new home. Vicki was learning about the things I liked and, early on, went out of her way to indulge me. This helped make me more comfortable and at ease. Everything was smooth, and for the most part, all was going smoothly in the beginning. Everyone put on a good face and set a good example. The ideal foster home you could say. I'm not saying it was all an act; it's just that over the years, there would be ups and downs, and the beginning definitely started off well. I got along well with the two youngest boys, David and Gregg, first. They would help me around the house or outside, and the three of us would often play with my ever-growing collection of Micro Machines. Mystic would join us, depending on what we might be doing, but half the time, it ended up with arguing. Kyle, on the other hand, kept to himself for the first month or two while I was there, but eventually, that wall came down too. Even though he was almost a year younger, he was different from me, because he had already outgrown toys and cartoons for the most part. I'll be honest; he still watched cartoons with me every now and then, but when you're in my position, entertainment and leisure can be somewhat limited, so that's what I chose. A few days before Christmas break, I took it upon myself to ask for a little spending money for school snacks and bought a candy bar or two every day. I used markers and drew lines over plain notebook paper for an artsy look, wrapped them, and took them home. It wasn't much, but I wanted to give everyone something for being so welcoming when I first moved in. Then just a few days before Christmas was the first annual Christmas season ritual, going to Grady's Christmas tree farm near Farmington. It was a family thing back then, and everyone came along. Those are the kind of memories I look back at fondly and cherish most. We got on the wagon, and it took us out to the trees until we found the perfect one. We cut it down and went back to the main area. By then, we were usually freezing our butts off and sometimes enjoyed hot apple cider before we headed home. The first year, we had trouble putting up the tree because it wouldn't fit in the tree stand. Ironically, that happened more than once in future years because we kept getting bigger trees.

I love the Christmas season. I just don't understand how some people can't appreciate the beauty and love of the holidays. A time you spend with family and create memories you wish you could revisit. I was able to have a few supervised visits with my mom and siblings. I remember showing Mom my new clothes and how nice I looked.

Then Mom gave me my Christmas present I had chosen, and she put on layaway just before I went into foster care in an attempt to patch things up from my birthday. As I opened it, I said, "More Legos?" Mom replied, "But I thought that's what you wanted." After I finished unwrapping, I realized it was the same pirate ship Lego set I had indeed chosen. I thought it was a different set entirely and that the ship was wrapped separately, thus that's why I said more Legos, plus the fact that I had been flooded with Lego sets in recent months. I wasn't disappointed at all, actually. Legos kept me occupied and held my interest at the time. Even my counselors from camp sent me a few fire department–themed Legos for Christmas. A few days before Christmas, my grandma and grandpa were supposed to stop by for a visit and give me my Christmas gifts. I had asked for a few things before I went into foster care but got an even bigger surprise I wasn't expecting. They were late to visit that day, and I immediately saw why my brother Victor was with them. It had been two years since I saw him last, and it seemed like forever. We talked about things a little bit, and he helped me unwrap the gifts I got from Grandma and Grandpa. That memory is a favorite of mine from those early foster care days. And I just now realized that was the last time my grandparents, Great-Grandma, Victor, and I would all be in the same photo.

As it would be every year after, after the holidays were a busy time. Thankfully, while I was still at school in Peoria, I got longer holiday breaks than the rest of the kids. The holidays always meant at least one party for Thanksgiving, usually at home or the place of Vicki's mom in Avon, and on Christmas, we normally went to her dad's for a pre-Christmas party, then her mom's, and then usually we stayed at home on the actual day. I did like Vicki's family mostly; her dad and stepmom were always friendly, and so were Vicki's brothers Brian, Greg, and Wally. Lee's family, on the other hand, was okay, but other than a few of his sons and two of his grandchildren, they didn't come around much. On Christmas Day, we all got up early to open our presents from under the tree. Needless to say, I got more Legos, which I asked for, and I remember a plushy from the *101 Dalmatians* cartoon. It was still popular at the time, and Dalmatians after all are the number-one fire department mascot. Diane and Bob came over later that day, and I got presents from them too, of course. Very strangely, of all the Christmases, that's the only one I don't remember what they gave me. It had already been a long day, but it was great just being with them for the holiday. We all have favorite holiday memories, but every time I think of the next one, I smile even though Kyle obviously wasn't too happy about it. Kyle, David, and I were all in our room, and David and I were playing with the Nerf air-powered missile launcher my grandparents gave me. David set it on the floor, stomped the rubber launch trigger, and it was launched just as Kyle looked up to be hit directly in the eye. Oh crap. Without blinking, David took off in an instant, and a pissed-off Kyle chased after him. That was before Kyle and I were friendlier with each other, but we look back at that moment now and just laugh.

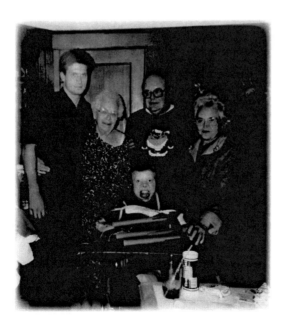

Chapter 17

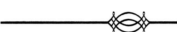

In January when the holiday magic had begun to wear off, I was finally headed back down Galveston. But it was my first trip down there with Vicki. As usual, I flew from Peoria to St. Louis and, from there, flew to Houston, where we were always greeted by Shriners and chauffeured down to Galveston. Every time we landed at Houston, I compared it to how a death row inmate felt walking the last mile. Nothing good awaited me, only pain and misery. It felt as if I had no control over my fate, because it was for my own good. Things were much different than the summer of 1991 and that round of surgeries. The new building made everything easier, and it was an altogether more comfortable atmosphere than the old hospital. And to top it off, the nurse whom I had so much trouble with before was no longer there, so that was one less thing for me to worry about. But unfortunately, she would soon be followed by my therapist Merilyn. She told me she was moving to Seattle, Washington, to work at a new hospital there and would no longer be my therapist. I wasn't thrilled with saying good-bye, but the other new change coming would at least make that easier. After this stay, I would be going to Shriners in Chicago for future clinical and surgical appointments. That meant no more long flights from Illinois to Texas or month-long hospital stays. And it would make hospital visits from family much easier. But before that could happen, I had to undergo the surgery I knew was coming months before. Merilyn and my doctors had told me back in the summer that they would eventually be performing an amputation revision on both of my legs. The surgery was needed because, after an initial amputation, the bone can continue to grow, especially on young amputees. Before my surgery, Pat Blakeney asked me, "Is there anything you need to make you more comfortable?" I told her about two requirements for my surgery. First and most importantly, I wanted to be asleep *before* they inserted that huge tube up my nose. That tube wasn't like a simple suction tube. It was large and painful, and it was inserted while using some kind of anesthetic gas. During the insertion, I couldn't breathe, and in my opinion, it was just needless torture. Second was the simple request of removing the urinary catheter before I woke up in the recovery room. It might seem like such a simple thing, but I always thought it was very uncomfortable, and not to mention awkward and embarrassing. And I despised the having that dang thing you-know-where.

Luckily for me, it all went just as I requested, and I was thankful for it, just two more things that made my stay that much easier on me. But what I wasn't expecting was the pain in my legs when I awoke in the recovery room. At first, the pain was mild, and I simply thought the bandages were wrapped too tight. There was always somebody nearby, and I told them the leg bandages were too tight and it was making them hurt. As with every surgery I ever had, my eyes were blurry and completely messed up, so I honestly can't tell if they physically did anything, but they still very much hurt, and the pain was worsening. And as usual, even though I'm trying to rest, I'm constantly asked, "Are you about ready to head back to your room, or we're almost ready to head back?" or any combination of ways emphasizing the fact. Even my most simple surgeries we're all-day affairs. I could go in at 9:00 a.m. and not be back in my room until midnight. But time is irrelevant when all of your senses are out of whack and you're in pain. Because I was still in pain when I finally got back to my room, I was given a morphine pump that had a self-dispense button I could hit with my elbow. I never had the option to self-medicate like that before. It helped the pain tremendously and allowed me to be comfortable enough to get some sleep. I remember it was Merilyn who eventually explained to me that the pain from the amputation revision was similar to having your legs broken and apologized for not saying anything about it beforehand. But then, before I was healed enough to get back in my chair, I was back under the knife for another neck release. I've lost count of how many of those I went through, but the process after the surgery started off with a bedridden week, and my head tilted up, and thus, I could only watch TV upside down for a few days. Compared to the bedridden months back in summer 1990 with no TV at all, it was just fine by me. Vicki was always present for surgeries and stuck around at least a few days afterwards but eventually always had to go home at some point. This meant I was alone. It wasn't so easy for me, but I managed to get by as I always did.

When I was finally back up and in my wheelchair, I had a few things to keep me occupied. Diane had mailed me a care package with candy, snacks, and Bon Jovi's newest album titled *Keep the Faith*, an appropriate title in my opinion. No matter what obstacles you face in life, you shouldn't give up, and at some point in our lives, we all need somebody to lean on. You must learn to ignore the hate and despair, hold onto your dreams, and *keep the faith*. I bided my time by learning the new lyrics or spending time in the playroom when I could. I also received a surprise letter from Kyle's friend Darrin Thurman. I met him when he stayed over during Christmas break, and the letter mentioned how he had fun with me the day we chased Mystic around the living room table. It was a simple letter, but it was cool of him to take the time to do so. It was nice to know I had positive impacts on people I barely know and that I'm in their thoughts when I'm so far away during my routine stays at the hospital. When Vicki returned, she brought a Gameboy that her brother Brian helped get me to give me something to do during those inevitable moments of boredom. It was nice to have those little distractions. Even the little things could make stressful hospital stays that much easier, because of the fact that I had two separate surgeries during that stay I was in Galveston for just over a month. Before I headed back home, the nurses and everyone held a small good-bye party, because this would supposedly be my last long term stay in Galveston. Cake and punch was served to staff and patients, pictures were taken, and it did indeed felt like the end of a chapter. I was going to a new hospital, and Merilyn was set to go in a new direction also. I would miss the friendships I had at Galveston, but it would be worth it if it meant being closer to home during surgeries and lengthy hospital stays. The release on my neck meant at least six months of wearing a neck brace. It was always uncomfortable, hindered my movement, and just plain ugly. It was yet another medical thing that set me apart and made me feel like a patient instead of just a regular teenager. I honestly think I hated that thing more than the face mask. As for my legs, when I headed back home, they still required daily wound care and wrapping. And because they were still healing, my legs also still had the stitches and staples in them and would be taken out when I went to the Shriners Hospital in Chicago for my first appointment there.

On our trip home, Vicki took the opportunity to tell me about a Peggy Harper, who was a volunteer with the Dream Factory in Pekin. The Dream Factory granted wishes to critically and chronically ill children around central Illinois. She had tried to find me months before, and she then saw me at the Christmas party of Vicki's dad. Vicki told me all about it and suggested I think about what I might want to ask for. When I got back home, I settled back into my routine albeit with the added pain in the butt, neck strap, and my legs still healing. Within a few weeks, I went up to Shriner's in

Chicago for my first checkup. That first trip up there was a long one, and it was the only time Lee ever accompanied me for anything medical. His work schedule is typically busier than Vicki's most of the year, but at the time, he was still off work due to the winter season. He worked in the construction industry, operating the big machines, and his days were always long, so when he was home, he tended to fall asleep when watching TV. Otherwise, his time was occupied by working on woodworking projects in his shop. Anyhow, we took the long route to Chicago by going through central Illinois, and I had my headphones on, listening to none other than Bon Jovi, of course. Upon arrival, the first thing I noticed was that right next to the hospital was an M&M/Mars candy factory. The only thing next to the Shriners in Galveston was more hospitals. The wait to see a doctor was stupidly long and boring. When I finally did see somebody, I was asked questions left and right about anything and everything. A lot of it was personal, and some of it, embarrassing. No offense to Lee, but it would have been easier having Vicki or Diane present for that stuff. My leg stitches and staples were finally taken out and rather painlessly, I might add, and I was grateful for that because I feared the pain that might come when they were finally removed. Then several hours later, we finally headed home until next time. I was starving for food that night, and we stopped at some random restaurant on I-80 near La Salle. By the time we got home, it was 1:00 or 2:00 a.m., and I was pretty much dead asleep in the van by then. Those days were simpler. I could fall asleep wherever and whenever without dealing with the scoliosis problems I endure now.

By this time, Kyle and I were no longer strangers to each other. We still shared the porch room, and it was around this time when we had our first confrontation, as you might call it. I won't go overly into details on Kyle or any of our many disagreements, but one day, for some reason, I don't remember why, but he got in my face, and I wouldn't back down. He threatened me, but I honestly was not scared. Yes, he could hit and physically hurt me, and I couldn't do anything in return, but I did not fear it. My perspective was simple—I had already been through and still faced more pain than I could receive from him. Nothing short of a shoulder punch and tons of name-calling and threats ever happened between us two, but that incident was the first. On the other hand, at least I knew I could count on him when we were out shopping and in public. I tended to ignore the rude stares and gawkers whenever I was out and about. But occasionally, there would be kids who went out of their way to follow us around. By then, Kyle had already warned them or would soon intervene. My favorite memory of Kyle taking action was during a trip to Walmart in 1995. Some kid who was clearly younger than us both was following us around the store, and even after he asked a question about what happened and if I could talk, he continued to pester us. Finally, Kyle had enough of it and told him, "Leave us alone, or I'll kick your ass." The kid laughed and said, "Yeah, right," and judged Kyle's age by his appearance as many people still do with me. Kyle told him he was fifteen and something else about being older than him. This kid didn't believe him, and so Kyle simply told the boy to ask me. My answer was "I am older than he is, and he *is* fifteen, and he *will* kick your ass." He finally got the hint and left us alone. So despite our occasional differences, he had my back in those situations.

After time thinking about it and a slight suggestion of something different from my first choice, I decided on a TV, VCR, and video camera from the Dream Factory, simply because having them would keep me occupied when I had nothing else to do. Initially, I wanted an electric guitar. Even though I knew I couldn't play one, I still thought it would be cool to own and at least mess around with. I was glad for the new TV and VCR because not only did it mean movies and my favorite shows, but it also gave me something to plug my Super Nintendo into, which I eventually got from my mom.

I remember March 9, 1993, fondly. I came home from school that day, expecting to celebrate David's birthday. Instead, I found Joey there waiting and curiously excited about something. Vicki told me I needed to take a quick shower because I was going somewhere, and it was Joey who spilled the beans during my shower when he said, "Where have you always wanted to go?" Within a guess or two, I said Bon Jovi? I was right, and immediately, my excitement level shot sky-high. Not only was I going to see Bon Jovi that night, but my counselors from camp were taking us to see his concert that night. It was a twofer as far as I was concerned, my first concert and another weekend in Chicago with my counselors. Before they arrived, I had Joey grab my Bon Jovi tape in hopes of getting it signed, and then we took off as soon as they arrived. I was too excited to rest despite my long day at school. But Joey actually slept half the way there. The concert was at what was then called Rosemont Horizon. The closer we got, it seemed as if every limo we saw might have the band in it. One of the things that stood out in Rosemont was the huge water tower with the rose mural painted on it. Every time I see it when driving on I-294, I think of my first concert that night. When we arrived at Horizon, we waited outside for what seemed like forever. It takes a lot to get me cold, but we were in line, and the temperature was cold enough that I was freezing, but it was worth it. When we finally got inside, the place was huge. Riggers and other workers were working till the very last second, getting everything ready. Then finally, the stadium was full, the lights were dimmed, and the band came out of an entryway directly underneath us, and we were seated just up and behind them. I did everything I could to get their attention, but with thousands of fans screaming, of course I was drowned out. Then the magic began as they rocked the crowd. I found myself just listening instead of singing along, as if to respect them and soak it all in. Mike Kilburg and Scott I know were with us that night, but I can't remember if LJ and Mike H. were too. The concert seemed to last forever, and it was about one thirty in the morning when we got to Scott's place and quickly to sleep. We didn't get to meet the band, but without their help, we wouldn't have been there in the first place. My first concert was awesome, and I owe it to those guys for their generosity and brotherhood.

That same weekend I was at the concert, unbeknownst to me, a hospital friend who worked with my school found a pregnant stray cat and took her in. I learned all about it later on and came home, asking if I could get a kitten. Due to past experience, when it involved potential pets, I was expecting the answer to be no. So I was pleasantly surprised when I was told yes. I planned everything ahead and got all the supplies I needed by the time I would bring my new cat home. I was told beforehand about their colors, and I decided on the one that seemed to match the colors of our orange-and-white cat Tommy we had from 1986 to 1989. On the day I was to bring him home, I brought along a pet taxi with me on the bus ride to school in Peoria. It felt weird bringing a pet carrier, but it wasn't that big of a deal, considering I was the only rider on the bus. At the end of the school day, I finally laid eyes on my new kitten, and he was so cute and small. I was ready to take him home for life with me, but that ride home was kind of tough. I could hear him crying and meowing in his cage as he stuck his tiny paws out. It made me feel bad for taking him away from everything he knew in his short life till then. But all the sadness was forgotten when I got home, and we quickly bonded. First off, we showed him his litter box and food bowl and let him adjust. I had been pondering his name for weeks until I got him, and while watching cartoons one day, I finally decided on the name Max. Max was the name of Goofy's son from Disney's *Goof Troop*. Max it seemed was full of energy as a kitten and, at times, just plain crazy, but that first evening, he fell asleep in a tiny ball next to my leg on my wheelchair. He took up no space on my lap at all, and that's when I knew the anguish during the ride from school was worth it and he was content to be with me. Max was everything I wanted in a cat and couldn't have asked for better.

A week or two after I brought Max home, Vicki and Lee were going out of town, and Bob and Diane were joining them. So Vicki had asked a friend to watch us. I was nervous as usual because somebody new would be helping me with my personal needs. Vicki reminded me that Charlene and Jessica would be there to help. But even that fact didn't really help much because they didn't assist me with my more private needs. It was only for two days at least. The lady watching us had two kids of her own who, prior to then, had not yet met me. I never know how some kids might react to meeting me, but her daughter, who I think was around eight or nine at the time, didn't seem bothered by my appearance. But on the first evening, I was simply messing around teasing and scaring her with a butter knife. I was just playing around as I had her cornered on the living room lounge seat, talking about eating her, and she's just laughing while she still kept her distance. At that point, I said, "Nah I think I'm going to go get my chainsaw." I turned around, went into my room, and that was supposed to be the end of it. Unfortunately, when I eventually came back out, I found out the poor girl thought I was serious and started crying while I was in my room. I didn't mean to scare her that bad. We are all teased by older individuals in our life at some point, and making her cry was truly not my intention. With the help of her mom assuring her I told her it was a joke, that I was sorry, I did not have a chainsaw, and she eventually was fine. The fun part of that weekend was when, out of sheer boredom, with the help of Kyle, Mystic, Gregg, and David, we played around with my new video camera for the first time. I honestly thought we might get in trouble for it when Vicki returned, but it was my camera, so she actually didn't care. I still have most of the home videos we made with that camera. But that weekend, we simply set up our bedroom like a concert and recorded me lip-synching to Bon Jovi. Gregg and David played guitar and piano while Mystic awkwardly danced behind us, and Kyle operated the camera until he switched places with Gregg. That same night, we made a small attempt at a home circus, albeit pathetic and embarrassing. But on a later date, when Max was still small, we recorded an improved version. And even though I've been warned to never post it publicly, such as on YouTube or *America's Funniest Videos*, it remains one of my favorite memories. We were all getting along with no arguing or fighting, and the finale was me doing another lip-sync to Bon Jovi's "Bed of Roses" and included everyone else just hanging out with me. But for this song, the lights were off, and we were using Kyle's black light for appearance and effect. Max was asleep in a ball on my lap, looking cute and peaceful, and all five of us had a rare moment of what I consider to be harmony. But it didn't last, with just one minute left until the song finished, the light came on, and Jessica burst in and said, "Time for bed." That disturbance didn't go well for Kyle, who immediately and angrily yelled, "F——!"

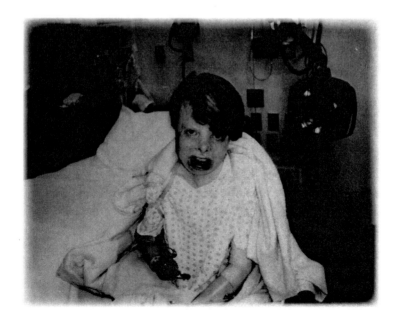

Chapter 18

With Easter also came the annual date Joey and I were burned, April 19. Our three-year mark like most came and went without celebration or much notice. We never dwelled on it, but it's always in the back of our minds. Diane gave me a newly reproduced Transformer I had wanted years before when Hasbro ceased production. She also gave me a set of *Star Wars* Micro Machines. Yes, I still collected them, but that specific gift sparked a new interest for me, which greatly intensified over time. After I opened the Micro Machines, Lee noticed a piece of paper inserted inside with an advertisement for the official *Star Wars Insider* magazine. Lee asked me if I would like a subscription. That surprises me even now because he never really expressed interest in such things, even saying, "I don't know why you watch this junk." But anyway, because he paid for my initial subscription, he was still a big factor toward me being the *Star Wars* fan I am now. I waited months until I received my first issue. Back then, it was four issues a year for $10. The months passed, and as I grew anxious, wondering when I would receive my first issue, Vicki sent a letter to them, explaining my unique situation. They mailed a personalized letter, apologizing for the slow response, and included a *Star Wars* Micro Machine set as a gift. My interest in *Star Wars* was just beginning.

I was still travelling to clinics in Chicago every few weeks or so, accompanied by a foster care social worker, Vicki, or another family friend. I found out sometime during those spring 1993 visits that the doctor's thought it would be too dangerous to do anything for my scoliosis for a few years while my body was still growing. I assumed a surgery would involve inserting a rod in my back or something like that. At the time, I still felt zero effects from my scoliosis and was still flexible enough I could actually rest my head on my knees during long car rides, albeit with a stiff neck, so having a foreign object permanently inside me just wasn't something I was comfortable with. Knowing what I know now if it could have been safely without risk, I probably would have done so. Anyway, back at home, I was officially settled in by then, but Max was still very much a kitten. He slept with me every night, and during those first few months, he would suck on my ear as I lay in bed trying to sleep. I didn't mind it, and his picture-perfect cuteness even earned him some TV time on WHOI 19 from Peoria when they asked for pet pictures to use during the weather forecast. The picture was of Max on my lap chewing on the straw in a cup I was holding. Both Lee and Vicki had many extended families because both were previously married and Vicki's parents were also. Vicki's brothers seemed a bit like my own uncles, probably more than they know. And I won't say much about her nieces. The older one from the very start seemed to have a rude attitude toward me because of my appearance. I remember one day her taunting me, calling me ugly as I went down the ramp outside. My only reply was, "I know," but I could hear Mystic defending me as I drove away down the sidewalk, trying to shrug it all off in my typical fashion. Lee, on the other hand, already had grandkids, and when I first met Dustin and his younger sister Ashley, it didn't go well for the latter. Ashley was still three or four when she met me, and unfortunately, she was the scared type. Every time I was near, she clung to Vicki's or Lee's legs, and I remember her crying one time she was alone in the kitchen and knew I was in the dining room. After that first visit, it was another two years or so before she came back. Dustin, on the other hand, started off as kind of a smartass little pest whom I teased a lot in the beginning, but he actually grew on me, and it seemed sometimes that he liked me more than I did him. On two occasions, I remember him crying because I wouldn't be home that weekend. One was for camp, and the other, I was staying at Diane's. He begged me to stay from camp, which wasn't going to happen, and then begged Diane to let him come with, so very clingy he used to be. Lee had two more grandsons, Randy and Marshall. Marshall had the same reaction as Ashley did, but unlike Ashley, he wasn't kept away from me until he was older. But with time, both would eventually get over their fears.

Sometime during early spring, the family went shopping for a spa. We all went to Peoria and checked out different models in a few stores. When Vicki and Lee finally chose one, it arrived on a flatbed, and the thing was so huge Lee needed serious help unloading it onto the concrete slab he had already poured himself. Bob arrived to help, as did a few others, and it was set in place. I think one of the first times I got in it was at Jessica and Charlene's birthday party—that was an experience. I felt like I was intruding on their fun, to be honest. It seemed like I was the awkward duck in the group, and as I sat in the spa, it was quiet, and I felt out of place. I don't remember when, but eventually over the summer, Lee built a huge patio deck around it. He was an excellent carpenter, and the first few months with them I had no idea how good he really was. His garage workshop would be the envy of any high school wood shop. He had anything and everything you would ever need for woodworking, and if he wasn't working, that's usually where you could find him. Those happy times during the first few months, when everyone got along without arguing and bickering, weren't to last, though. Every family has squabbles and grief of some sort, and we would be no exception. Gregg and David had their brotherly fights, Kyle and Mystic, Mystic and Jessica, Charlene and Kyle, and any other combination. But in a foster home, sometimes that rivalry is intensified with the non-foster children fighting for attention among each other and the foster siblings. This led to Kyle getting in more trouble than any of them, simply because of his temper problem, which easily and too often became physical. But one of the first incidents that showed me a darker side of things was when Charlene ran away. I still don't fully understand why she left, and I barely remember the details from the night before. I think it was something about not being allowed to go out with a boyfriend and maybe an argument about it, but she was gone the next morning, and I haven't seen or heard from her since. I was surprised because out of all them, even me perhaps, she seemed the most behaved and well adjusted. After all, she liked it there enough to take Davis as her adopted name. She wouldn't be the last to leave, though—that's for sure. More than I can remember ran away over the years, but Charlene was the only one I would have never expected to.

I was still having occasional visits back in Monmouth with Mom and my siblings almost once a week. Most of the time, it annoyed me, because all I wanted to do after a long day at school was chill out. I had been trying for weeks to convince Mom to let me bring my cockatiel Duncan back to Vicki and Lee's, but she refused. This in turn just pissed me off, because I was being kept from something that belonged to me, and I felt was my right to have. So throughout one particular visit, I made it known he belonged to me and it just wasn't fair. Finally, she gave in, and I took him back with me. When we returned to Rapatee, Max was outside and immediately saw Duncan's cage sitting on the ground while I was helped out of the car. Max immediately took the opportunity to run circles around the cage, trying to get his prize, and all the while, Duncan was flapping around in sheer terror. I'm surprised he didn't have a heart attack and Duncan's antics only magnified Max's interest. Eventually, Max would realize he was off limits, and I was even able to place Duncan on Max's back without worrying about him ending up as his dinner. We were occasionally training new nurses to replace others and break up the shifts so any one nurse wasn't coming in too often repeatedly. But there was always a few that, for whatever reason or another, I just didn't care for. There was one in particular the first few months in foster care who seemed to rush at her job and do everything half-assed. I'd rather have somebody slow than one who rushed and didn't do the job right the first time. Another nurse whose name I also don't remember decided one evening after my shower to carry me all the way from the bathroom to my bedroom instead of using my wheelchair. She picked me up under both arms with the towel draped only over my front and carried me out one door leading to Jessica's room through the living room, where *everyone* was, into the dining room, and finally into my bedroom. I valued my privacy, and needless to say, I was pretty pissed off that she dared violate my dignity like that. Just because I'm disabled and in a wheelchair doesn't mean it's all right to be paraded naked in front of everyone like that. We deserve the same respect and privacy as anyone else. I did get revenge on her at least with the help of Duncan. She was terrified of birds, and I had him on my shoulder one day as I came in behind her while she was cornered in my room. Her reaction was priceless. She freaked out, begging me to keep him away, as if yelling, "Bloody murder!" I really found it hard to comprehend how anyone could be scared of a little ol' bird. It wasn't long after that she stopped coming around. So I guess one little bird was too much for her.

Before the end of the school year was the annual Lindbergh Middle School Athletics Competition, and not long after that was the seventh-grade field trip to the capitol house down in Springfield. That was the first time I ever visited Springfield, and it was cool to see the history. Even though I didn't have as much interest and appreciation of history as I do now, it wasn't ever a subject I hated like math. When we visited the capitol building and reached the upper floor of the dome, my fear of heights tried to take over. It really bugs me how it can bother me now, but when I was young, I used to love climbing the trees and being up high. But being in a wheelchair is a world away from that. It's as if being able-bodied meant that I had full control, which meant I had nothing to fear. I'd never fall or get hurt, and being in a wheelchair is the opposite—always at risk and out of my control. I don't have hands to grasp or brace, so whatever happens will happen so to speak. We didn't get to see the governor, but I do remember a picture taken of the entire seventh-grade class in the house senate, though I don't know what happened to it. At the end of the year were the school ceremony and achievement awards. I received another reward for being one of the top readers in school. I was always proud of the fact that I was one of the top readers, because I had never been one of the best at anything and I was finally acknowledged for excelling at something academically. I guess the long bus rides I had gave me a time advantage. Later on even in high school, I tended to finish chapters or entire books before the required date, but my English grades didn't exactly reflect that fact.

Before summer arrived, Kyle switched rooms, so Gregg and David were then sharing the porch room with me. My first summer in Rapatee was awesome. I think that one was one of my busiest during the earlier years in foster care, so overall, the boredom wasn't too bad. For weeks, I had been looking forward to the awesome new dinosaur movie *Jurassic Park*. I had always liked dinosaurs, and the special effects were supposed to blow your mind away by letting audiences see and experience them in a way never seen before. Father's Day was around the same time as the movie release that year, and while shopping at Kmart in Galesburg, I noticed a sign out front asking kids to write a little something about Father's Day. The winner would receive four gift certificates to nearby Sirloin Stockade and a $25 gift certificate to Kmart. It had a five-hundred-word require-ment, so I figured, why not give it a try? When I got home, I wrote a few things about Bob. I mentioned the ride he gave me on his ATV a few weeks prior and how in a way he was like my dad. He just kind of assumed that role without asking or thought of reward. A few days later, we got a call saying my essay had won the Father's Day contest. I was surprised I had actually won, and I gave the gift certificates to Vicki, Lee, Bob, and Diane so the four of them could go out to dinner. And I was allowed to spend the gift certificate at Kmart, which I used to buy the *T. rex* from *Jurassic Park*. That movie began, yet another interest for me. Like I said earlier, I already liked dinosaurs before then, but the toys that came with that movie had a level of detail way better than older dinosaur toys. When *Jurassic Park* was finally in theaters, I was begging to go see it every time we were in town. Surprisingly though, it was actually my grandparents who finally did take me to see it. My grandma was worried it was going to be scary and, for some reason, was suspicious I might have seen it already. I had not seen it yet, and I actually would have told her if I did, but because of previews and the toys I had, parts of the movie, and plot had been spoiled, and I could sense when a charac-ter was about to meet their fate. I said something like, "That guy is going to die," to which Grandma replied, "Are you sure you haven't seen this?" Both she and Grandpa jumped once or twice during the movie, and the first time watching a movie like that is memorable. It had groundbreaking special effects, and it truly brought dinosaurs to life on screen as if they were real. I still get the chills when I hear the *T. rex* thumping and that unmistakable roar. After the movie, we went to Walmart, where they bought me a few *Jurassic Park* toys. Most of my interests came and went. I will always like dinosaurs. To some extent, my *Jurassic Park* fever got pretty intense for a while, but eventually, it faded, and *Star Wars* would forever dominate my destiny.

Chapter 19

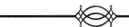

Heavy rain throughout the Midwest early that summer brought the great flood of 1993. Everybody who was around back then can still remember the extent of the flooding and how bad it was. The mighty Mississippi was the most affected, but numerous smaller rivers were also past flood stage. Prior to then, I had never seen flooding up close and personal. During the height of the local flooding, we went to London Mills, where I saw the fields north and south of town underwater and volunteers preparing sandbags to protect their properties and the downtown area. I told Vicki I wish there was some way I could help, even though by then they were almost finished with the sandbagging process. For weeks, every time the news was on, you could see the stories about the flooding all the way from Minnesota down to Missouri. Weather forecasters said it would be weeks and even months until it all receded, and that's when Vicki told us we might miss what would be my first trip to Six Flags. The flooding was so bad in the St. Louis area that it might prevent us from going. That news was disappointing to hear, because it was a trip I looked forward to. Fortunately, I didn't hear no for an answer, and the trip was still a go. I remember spending the night at Bob and Diane's the night before, and I was absolutely too excited to sleep. I didn't want to go to bed, but back then, I rarely had a choice in the matter.

Bob and Lee were both staying home to work, and it was Vicki and Diane who were taking a van full of seven on the trip. For Diane, that would be the only time she did so for the simple fact that so many kids drove her crazy.

On the long ride to St. Louis, we stopped at Springfield for breakfast when Gregg and David were fighting. On any long ride with kids, squabbles and arguments are inevitable, and Vicki threatened to leave them in Springfield, where Lee was supposedly working at the time, but it didn't happen. As we got closer to the Mississippi River near the St. Louis area, we started to see the major flooding we saw on TV. The local flooding at home was nothing compared to the scale down there. Upon seeing the initial flooding as we got closer, I honestly had doubts about whether we would reach our destination, but our first tourist stop was at the Gateway Arch in St. Louis. The Mississippi had come all the way up to the steps leading down to a river front area near the arch, and again, the extent of the flood just boggled the mind. As usual, I was in my manual wheelchair, and as I looked down, I felt very nervous by how close I was to those steps. Once again, it's a feeling of control; it would only take a momentary second for my chair to start rolling, and at the time, I couldn't stop it if did so. We left the steps to get ready to go up the arch, and I calmed down for the time being. I must admit the arch looks and feels so much bigger in person than it does in pictures. Standing next to either end on the ground, you can't help but feel so small compared to it. My expectations of the ride up consisted of getting inside a trolley/booth and riding it all the way to the top without getting out. I thought the booth would go all the way up to the viewing windows and simply come back down, but unfortunately for my fear, I was mistaken. Diane was absolutely terrified of heights even more so than I was, so I don't know why she was fine up there. I didn't have my wheelchair, and thus, I was picked up and sat right in front of the window. The view was cool, but that same fear I felt at the top of John Hancock Tower in Chicago had different opinions. The closer I was to that window, the more nervous I was, and I was already as close as I could physically get. Needless to say, I was glad when we returned to ground level, and from there, we headed west to our next stop, the St. Louis Science Center. We didn't spend a lot of time there, but at the *Triceratops* fossil restoration exhibit, the lady working on it gave me a small piece of the skull, which I still have in its tiny Ziploc bag. From there, we headed even further west to Jellystone campground near Six Flags. The campground was neat, and it had modern amenities, like an arcade, swimming pool, and shower. But I was still having two showers a day, and even then, there would be no exception. It wasn't so bad, except I tended to be itchy afterward, and in the evening, I was made to wear a robe while it was still daylight, and everyone else was still in normal clothes. This irritated the heck out of me because I didn't like being treated differently in such a way that the other kids didn't have to. I protested the idea months before, but it fell on deaf ears. "Oh sure, everyone wears pajamas or robes at this time of day," I was told. Who was it, may I ask? I never did find out. The other part that sucked about it was getting dressed and my daily care in the cabin. I didn't like the others around when I was mostly naked while my daily care was being done. All the kids went outside, except Kyle, who thought the unspoken rule and request didn't apply to him, nor did he care sometimes.

The first evening at the campground, we could see and faintly hear the fireworks gong off at Six Flags, and once again, I was begging to go that night. I was told we would have all day tomorrow at the park, so good things come to those who wait. "But I want it NOWWWWW." That night I thought it unusual that I found myself shivering, but I was more annoyed by Vicki, Diane, and Jessica trying to play a prank on Gregg and David. David was in the bunk above Gregg, and they were trying to pour water on Gregg to make him think David wet the bed above him. I told them to be quiet and turn the damn flashlight off, but I was just told to shut up. "Give me a break. I was trying to sleep. How rude can you get?" I don't think Gregg fell for it, though. The next morning, I was refreshed and ready to go. Only once before my burns had I ever been to any theme park, and that was Silver Dollar City back in 1987. Back then, I had gone with my grandparents and Victor to Branson, Missouri. That was a memorable weekend aside from the pontoon "duck" ride when I was dying of thirst and then feeling sick that night. Now with my burns, the only downside was the crowds and the staring that came with them. But at least I was able to bypass lines, and because of the fact that I was limited to rides I could ride safely and comfortably, I went on those rides repeatedly. It was summer after all, but luckily, I was able to stay cool enough by alternating between water rides and indoor attractions such as the stage shows. Almost immediately after getting inside the park, I remember Jessica told me to hold her cigarettes. I wasn't responsible for her belongings, and I never appreciated being treated like a shopping cart or a purse. If I remember correctly, they fell, were lost among the huge crowd, and I could have cared less. It simply wasn't my job to babysit their belongings. Holding the purse or bag of the person pushing my wheelchair on the other hand is entirely different, giving me something to watch while they go off and do whatever is another. One of the first rides I went on was the log flume, but like the tidal wave, I only went on it once. The height combined with the sudden deceleration wasn't very enjoyable for me, especially the latter. When I rode the tidal wave upon hitting the water, I slid forward fast and hard enough to bump my leg stumps on the front of the ride. I did enjoy getting soaked on the bridge above it, but I must say, even that part was pretty intense. The wave hit hard enough to flip my chair over if nobody were around to brace it. I didn't ride any roller coasters, with the exception of one smaller slower one Vicki duped Diane and me into riding. The speed nor height wasn't too bad for me, but it was enough that I wasn't comfortable with how much movement and how insecure I felt in the seat. I had no belt on just Diane's arms and the guard bar that came down in front of us. But I felt like I was all over that seat, flopping back and forth. My favorite ride by far was Thunder River, and I quickly realized it was just a floaty secure ride and I didn't have to worry about flying out of my seat or coming to a sudden stop or deceleration. The ride was made to seem tense as if you're always going to crash, and I always got wet on that ride. I always rode it twice in a row, which only helped guarantee I was soaked before I got off. That first year, I remember we saw at least two shows. One was a prop comedy that I don't remember, and the other was the *Robin Hood: Prince of Thieves* stunt show. I particularly liked this one because I had read a very good older book about Robin Hood during school that year. I was able to sit right up front closer to the action, and the only thing missing was a free roasted turkey leg one of the stage actors randomly handed out to the crowd. Overall, it was a great first visit to the park and a perfect way for kids to de-stress during the summer. On our trip back home, we made one more stop, and that was the St. Louis Zoo. We saw just a small handful of exhibits, but the one that stood out most to me was the bird house. In a huge part of it, the birds were allowed to fly free over your head, and there were signs advising visitors to be careful with fingers. We would have stayed longer, but when we tried to board the train to ride around the zoo, for some reason, supposedly because of my disability, we were denied. I was disappointed with the decision to leave so soon, but refusing our ride on the train cut short our visit, and from there, we headed back home.

Not much later after our trip that summer, I found out my mom was in the hospital after some sort of breakdown, and my siblings were scattered among Kirk and relatives for the time being. When I visited her in the hospital, I told her about my trip to St. Louis, and as usual, it was like no big deal to her. She just never seemed enthusiastic and interested when I told her stuff like that back then. But I guess you could say she was distracted by her situation at the time. When I visited Joey, he told me he was staying with Kirk, and I told him to get out of there if he ever needed and to call the police if Kirk ever tried anything. I might have been slightly overreacting, but without Mom there to keep Kirk from going overboard, who knows. Heck, Kirk once told me himself in these exact words that my mom kept him from doing anything or he'd go to jail. I don't remember how long Mom was in the hospital, but summer was speeding by fast, and quickly approaching was my second year at burn camp.

Chapter 20

Camp once again was around the end of August about two weeks, before school started. Everything leading up to it was pretty much the same, except for the simple fact that I was in foster care this time around. Vicki drove me to the Galesburg Fire Department, where I met up with Joey, and from there, we went to Moline, where we picked up another camper. Jimmy Palmer was still with us, and I think that year was the first-year Bomber, a.k.a. Justin Williams, joined us. I was very excited to get to camp, but it quickly turned to embarrassment when literally everyone was screaming and cheering as I entered the lodge. I was happy to be there, but you don't necessarily love that kind of attention when you're thirteen and especially when quiet and shy as I was. All the guys from the previous year were back, and that year, our cabin was Black Oak. I had hoped for the same counselors, because obviously that would be easier for everyone involved. A major difference that year was I remembered to bring along my eating device. That meant no more embarrassment of being fed and made mealtimes more enjoyable. We enjoyed a lot of the activities from the previous year, including muckman suitcase, capture the flag, and the puppet show. The one all-camp activity they never skipped over the years was the dance. Rain or not, it always went on, with the only exception of tornado threats in later years. That year though, we had a special daytime performance by a Chicago area Michael Jackson impersonator. Joey and I were near the lodge entrance when we saw Rona Roffey, the camp director, drive up with him seated in the golf cart. Joey immediately said while freaking out, "It's Michael Jackson." I, on the other hand, knew it wasn't him, because he had lost the dark skin tone sometime back in the '80s. Despite his skin being darker than the real Jackson, he was actually pretty good. And initially, Joey wasn't the only one to be fooled thinking he was the real thing.

Camp '93 was the first year I wasn't the only camper in a wheel-chair. That year, a younger camper named Nathan Boston was in Joey's cabin. Nathan was in a wheelchair due to spina bifida. And over the years, he wouldn't be the only one. It made me wonder why having spina bifida could lead to burns and the fact that each spina bifida camper was also black. But that year, we both rode on top of the same fire truck during the visitors' day parade, and we were also able to enjoy something set up just for the two of us. A few of the counselors had rigged up a kind of zip line on the hillside specially meant for our wheelchairs. I was obviously nervous but willing to try with encouragement and thorough description of how it would be done. I remained in my chair while straps were fastened and wrapped around it until it was secure, then I was hoisted about eight to ten feet up into the air, and while maintaining comfortable speed and control, I was led down the hill where I came to a gentle landing on the ground. It was easy as pie and definitely made us feel more special, because it was something just for the two of us in wheel-chairs. While at camp that year, I realized that I was developing a skin problem. During my Six Flags trip, it started as unusual chills that first night trying to sleep. On the evening of Sports-O-Rama, those unusual chills came back, and I was shivering. The weather wasn't hot, but it wasn't really cold enough to make me shiver either. I wasn't sick or anything, but at the time, I didn't know that. I felt fine other than the fact that my shivering had no explanation. And it would be months later until I had an explanation for it. There were still moments I overheated and even required assisted cooling, usually by a water hose, but it wasn't too often. That year, I also brought along my video camera so I could show everyone back at home how fun camp was. Scott Vaughn brought his along too, and between the two of us, we recorded a few hilarious moments. The first one, which I still sometimes think about sending into *America's Funniest Videos*, is of Mike Kilburg having trouble on the high ropes plank bridge section. He had himself positioned awkwardly and was having trouble advancing, all the while Dave Poore was laughing his ass off behind the camera. The other was during the puppet show when a huge dog costume of *Sesame Street* quality entered the lodge and Rona's dog freaked out, barking at the intruder. Rona tried to hush her, but in the end, she wound up on the back of the costume with eyes wide open, as if she saw a ghost. I was surprised she didn't pee all over the costume in terror. It was great hanging out with my group again. Only once a year did I get that opportunity to truly hang with guys my own age on equal terms. Once again, I must point out the bond I have up there doesn't exist anywhere else. I simply didn't have the friendships at home that I did at camp. On the second to last day, a visitor stopped by camp who worked for the company which produced Bon Jovi's music. Somebody had told them about me being a fan, and I was given a brand-new Sony CD Walkman and a sampling of new CDs, one being Bon Jovi's *Keep the Faith* album. But that wasn't all. I was also given a picture of the band and a signed copy of the *Keep the Faith* album cover. I was overly excited and again surprised by the generosity shown to me by people I've never met. And even though I didn't see the band personally sign it, I hoped and believed it was still authentic. Before I knew it, the week was quickly over, and it was time to head back home. Back then, time seemed to fly faster, and even though I don't mention every little tiny detail from camp, keep in mind that I never missed a single year at camp, and those earlier years were twenty years ago. So details and memories from those earlier years aren't as numerous, but I never forget the various special moments from year to year. Camp will always have a special place in my heart. I've always held the belief that for a burn survivor, the healing never truly ends. We face challenges and miseries throughout life, and the compassionate support at camp is something I couldn't live without. When campers arrive on the first day, many hid their scars with long sleeves, but as the week progressed, we don't even notice them. The worst thing when you are a kid is being and/or thinking you're different. The trouble come from the fact that in school being different often made you a target. So by the time another school year ends, I was always ready for the rejuvenation I got at camp. I was always refueled, ready, and raring to go with the positive energy and self-esteem boost from camp.

The ride home that year seemed quieter than the previous. We were all sad to go and tried to hide our emotions as we watched a movie that was on the van's small TV. It was pointless to hide though, because our emotions were clearly obvious to one another. After getting back to Galesburg, Joey went his way while I went mine, and camp 1993 was the first time I had been away from home since going into foster care. That first year, Vicki had lots of questions about camp, such as, "Did you have fun?" "Did you get her postcard?" and "Did you behave yourself as suggested on the card?" It was actually quite the opposite, because that year I was in the burping contest during muckman suitcase, and even though I didn't win, I came second, and that was without the aid of a soda. At the end of the week during cabin awards, I was given the internal gastric propulsion technician award. *Belch*, excuse me. I was tired and worn out when I got home, so I didn't really do much. That special time of year had come to an end, and I found myself back at school again. It was the beginning of eighth grade and my last year at Lindbergh

Middle School. Before the year was over, I had to make a decision on where I was going to attend high school the next year. But for the time being, I was stubbornly insistent on sticking with my classmates from Lindbergh. My first day back that year was actually the first time I was present on the first day of school. The awkward result was I did not know which homeroom I had, and I felt like an idiot awkwardly wandering the halls. I think it was Mr. Simpson who ended up telling me I had Mrs. Rynearson that year. Mr. Simpson was cool; he wasn't exactly a teacher himself, and he could pal round with the students in almost an older brother way. At least that's how he was with me. At home, the start of the school year eventually brought new shows, and in September, I was caught by surprise how much I enjoyed a new cartoon called *Animaniacs*. I don't know why I found the show so hilarious, but I always thought the catchy music was what attracted me to it initially. But seriously though, even watching the show twenty years later, it makes me wonder how kids watched that stuff. There's so much subtle humor a kid never picks up on, and I still find puns I never noticed before. I loved the show so much I got some blank video tapes, and every day after getting home from school, I recorded every previously unrecorded episode. Some people just never grow out of cartoons, and I honestly don't see why you have to. Youth is something that should be cherished and held on to. If you enjoy something, it makes you happy, and it's not hurting anyone, then by all means, keep enjoying it. Who cares what others think. Rob Paulsen voiced three of the main characters, Yakko Warner, Dr. Scratchansniff, and Pinky on that show, and his quote is a life philosophy to live by: "Laughter is the best medicine, and the cool thing is you can't OD and the refills are free." Truer words are indeed rarely spoken. Laughter turns negative into positive, heals the mind and soul, and brings darkness to light. In my situation, humor has and always will be an important aspect of life that keeps me going. Laughter is a gateway and a stepping stone to happiness.

When something ruins your day, sometimes all you can do is laugh it off and move on. I also have my own quote that never fails to put a smile on my face. "Confucius says, 'He who no laugh at fart isn't human.'" Okay, it may be crude potty humor, but I bet if you're reading this right now, you at least chuckled and/or smiled to yourself, which was my intention.

Early October meant two things, my birthday and the annual Spoon River Drive. Rapatee was on the route, and that meant tons of traffic during the first two weekends of October when it's held. Prior to that year, I had never really known what the drive was all about. It started simply as an annual scenic drive enjoying the fall foliage in towns from southern Knox County down into Fulton County, and that's all I assumed it to be. But over the years, it evolved to include roadside stands, flea markets, and craft markets, which sprouted up from Knoxville down south to Lewistown. It still attracts people from all over the country every year. My first scenic drive while in Rapatee, we got up early because we were having a yard sale. I was getting rid of some older junk of my own, but the early October morning was cold, and I never enjoyed getting up early. Lots of folks came through Rapatee, and even my grandma and grandpa stopped by on their route. On October 4, while sitting outside watching people come and go, Vicki whispered to me about a joke to play on Diane. Diane was with us that day because we were all going to Chuck E. Cheese's for my birthday that night. When Diane had her back turned, Vicki placed fake poop on my wheelchair's lap board then walked away. Diane came back over, and I gave her a fake look of disgust and said, "Max crapped on my lap board." Inside, I was laughing my ass off, and I could see in Diane's face she was disgusted. She got a piece of toilet paper, and as she picked it up, she noticed instead of squishy and gooey, it was hard and rubbery. I was laughing as Vicki came out of the porch room. My first birthday in foster care was a big deal at Chuck E. Cheese's. At fourteen years old, I might have been a little old for it, but Kyle seemed to enjoy it just as much as I did, so go figure. For me, going there was mostly a pizza thing and the fact that as a kid I had only been there twice before I was burned. Bob, Diane, and my grandparents were all there to celebrate my birthday as well. Before we had cake, Diane actually shoved part of it in my face, trying to relive the moment when I shoved my own face in the cake years before at Methodist, and then came my birthday presents. Diane and Bob gave me the reproduced Optimus Prime I had begged for back in the spring. Finally, I had an Optimus Prime to call my own after the traumatic day back in kindergarten long ago. My grandma gave me some more *Star Trek* stuff, which I had been interested in since the previous Christmas, and of course, I got Micro Machines of various types. It was definitely a great birthday that year. My mom had got me cake the year before, but the neighborhood kids freeloading back then didn't exactly qualify as a party.

I continued with visits at home, but gradually, they shifted from taking place at Monmouth to the Catholic Social Services (DCFS) building in Galesburg. Mom mentioned around that time that she realized the state planned to keep me in foster care until I was at least eighteen. And she obviously was not happy about it. I compared her anger to how she reacted when my grandparents wanted to keep Victor until he graduated or when she supposedly heard Kirk wanted to take us kids away back in the late '80s. Things were slowly falling apart for my mom, though it wasn't necessarily Kirk who seemed to be the problem by then. During one particular visit at home, I remember Joey mention Mom had to steal food from the store. That's when I knew things weren't so good. I always assumed me being gone only increased financial strain without the aid of my social security assistance. And Kirk, I assume, was no longer supporting financially. An unemployed single parent just can't take care of four kids alone.

My school picture from eighth grade in my opinion looked terrible. My skin by then was severely red and blotchy, and we just couldn't figure it out. It was itchy and even drained fluid in tiny amounts. I hated it, not only because of how it felt but also because of how it made me look. Thanksgiving that year was the usual; I split it between going to Bob and Diane's and then with everyone else at Vicki's mom's in Avon. Though I honestly preferred Thanksgiving at the Wells' because I was more comfortable there. It was less crowded, easier for my wheelchair, better food, and I could also spend the night. To me, Thanksgiving meant turkey, and at the Wells, I knew I could get my fix. Nothing against Vicki's mom, Elaine, back then; I just still wanted to spend time with Bob and Diane that holiday without the chaos. I'm not sure when, but sometime during that winter season, I went with Vicki to visit Peoria Central High School. I was still set on staying in Peoria, but everyone involved was insistent that I explore and consider my options before making a choice. Mr. Noble, who was a teacher at Lindbergh the previous spring, gave us a tour. Already I saw one positive for staying in Peoria. I enjoyed Noble's class the year before and thought he was cool partly because I remember him talking about being in the navy. But now that I think about it, I also realize Mr. Noble was one of my first male teachers other than my music or PE teachers years before. During my tour, I also saw a few of my former classmates who had moved on from Lindbergh, yet another reason to choose Peoria. But the place was huge, crowded, and chaotic, and that made me feel uneasy. Still, for the time being, I remained focused with staying in Peoria. Kyle and Jessica both wanted me to choose Valley, so my Christmas break was when I followed Kyle for a day at Spoon River Valley High School. My visit to Central may have occurred before or after, but I know my visit at Valley was during my holiday break because Kyle's classes were preparing for the holiday with parties. In particular was watching Prancer in Mrs. Boughton's room. The biggest negative if I chose Spoon River basically was starting again in a new place like I had so many times before. Going to Central might be a new building with new teachers and new nondisabled classmates, but all if not most of my current classmates would be there with me. I saw a few advantages to attending Valley, though first of all it was nowhere as huge and crowded as Central. Second was the big reason for choosing Valley, and that was the fact that my cousin Nick was there also. During lunch, Nick sat with us, and I immediately thought how easier it would be with his support and to be able to hang with him at lunch every day. I felt welcomed that day, and Kyle actually held back the typical teasing I sometimes got from him. He had also told me I would have no trouble with anyone during my visit. Toward the end of the day, though, I did get bored in one of his classes and stole his pencil. I was messing around and didn't give it back until his teacher Mrs. Gurgurich told me to do so. Also, choosing Valley would mean no more predawn waking up for school to ride thirty-five miles one way. I was no longer dead set on going to Central in Peoria. After visiting Valley, I seriously pondered the pros and cons of each school.

The holidays that year were even busier than the year before. Those early years, it seemed we had more parties to attend. We went to the annual Christmas party held by Catholic Social Services in Galesburg. That was a large gathering of all the foster families in the Knox county area, which consisted of the usual gifts and food. That year was also the first year we went to the Dream Factory Christmas party in Pekin. All the kids who had received wishes over the years were welcome, as well as their families, but that first year it was just Jessica who came along. I always felt too old going to that particular party, especially as I got older, yet they said I was still welcome no matter how old I get. I liked going, because it was a holiday party and it was something festive to do, but too often some of the volunteers tended to treat me younger than I was. It still happens every now and then, but I tolerate it for the most part. Then there were the family parties. We rarely went to any of Lee's family for any holiday. They might stop by and say hello or visit with them on non-holidays, but we always seemed to stick with Vicki's family. At the place of Vicki's dad in Pekin that year, I was annoyed I was given a pack of Matchbox cars. I know it might sound greedy or selfish, but I was only annoyed because mine seemed more childish compared to Kyle's, and keep in mind he's actually younger than I am. So to me, it just didn't seem fair. But I ended up pleasantly surprised when he presented me a homemade cat condo for Max. After that, the simple Matchbox cars made sense, and the condo was almost overkill, but Max loved it. We also went to the Christmas party in Avon with Vicki's mom, Elaine. Once again, some unfairness reared its head. Initially, I don't remember what I received, but Kyle got a card with cash, as did his cousins close to our age. I only got frustrated because I wanted to be treated equally because we were all about the same age, give or take a year or two. Vicki ended up whispering, and I got a card with cash, and after that, there were no further misunderstandings. Like I said, it's not greed; I would have been fine if we had all been given toys or whatever. I just didn't like being treated younger and differently than those my age who were also given gifts.

That year was the only year we all went up to my grandparents for a Christmas party while in foster care. The whole family coming along, including Bob and Diane, was almost as good as my favorite holiday memories during the mid '80s. Those years when everyone on my dad's side was gathered together are among my favorite Christmas memories from my childhood. As usual, we had dinner, complete with all the fixings, and the younger kids always ate at the kids' table. For some reason, it was always Grandma's scalloped corn that I seem to remember enjoying most. Looking back, I think it was because hers was the best and I didn't have it that often from anyone else. After dinner, we went into the living room as our family used to do back when I was younger, only this time Grandpa wasn't in his Santa suit and the simple fact that it was a different family now. I was given some more Micro Machines and *Star Trek* stuff, and everyone else also received gifts from my grandparents that day. As a special gift, my grandma even framed the Father's Day essay I wrote for Bob and gave it to them. I spent Christmas Eve overnight with Bob and Diane. The night before, I could see all the gifts under their small tree and begged to open just one. Surprisingly, they agreed to let me open one, but ironically, it was a *Jurassic Park* figure I already had, so obviously I had to wait until I could unwrap the others the next day. On Christmas Day, Vicki, Lee, and everyone else came to Bob and Diane's for Christmas lunch. Out of all our holidays over the years, that time was the only one that I spent the night then had everyone at the Wells on Christmas Day. I guess transporting everyone and Diane's work schedule changed things up from year to year. So fitting everybody's schedules and time windows wasn't always easy. I had high hopes for two particular gifts that year. One was the *Jurassic Park* compound, which I could play with Gregg and David to satisfy those destructive urges. It was a huge compound that could be ripped and torn apart by the dinosaurs from the movie. I even ended up making a short home movie with Max tearing it up. But due to no motivation on Max's part, it was a dud. Check out Jurassic Cat on Youtube. The other I hoped to and did receive was a Sega Genesis. I don't really know why I wanted to change from Nintendo to Sega, but I think the better game selection and easier control pads were important factors to switching game systems. Diane told me she got a deal on QVC, and it included two controllers, Sonic 1 and 2, and even a guidebook for beating the game. Needless to say, I was satisfied, and some might say spoiled. That year, you would probably be right because even I think too much might have been spent on me that year with just those two pricey gifts. Not long after everyone had opened gifts and everyone was winding down from dinner and gift opening, my teenage excitement was still rising. Months of eagerly anticipating my new Sega Genesis admittedly took over, and in my excitement, I shamefully said, "Come on, let's go. I want to get home and play my Sega." Bob heard it, and I immediately realized I sounded too greedy and selfish during a momentary lapse of judgment. Other than that nasty little moment, that year was my favorite Christmas with Bob and Diane. It was a time when everyone was gathered around, and we were still young enough to feel the holiday excitement and magic only felt in your youth. I still love Christmas, and it's my favorite time of year, but as I got older, I just didn't feel the same magic as when I was younger.

After the New Year, Vicki and Lee were set to go on a Caribbean cruise to celebrate their wedding anniversary, and if I remember correctly, I think it was before I went back to school, because I know their actual anniversary was late December. Fortunately for me, Diane and Bob were staying with us to help me and watch us all still at home. But unfortunately for me, though, the day we went to the airport to see them off, I began to feel sick. I don't get sick often, but on the ride back home from the airport, I felt miserable. Diane attempted to rub my head to make me feel better, and to be honest, it did help me relax. I admit I was always a sucker for head rub. But I don't think I was sick long because I don't recall being sick for a lengthy amount of time or missing any school days. Just a year before, I was in Galveston for the surgery on my legs and my neck release, and I was still going to the Shriners clinic in Chicago, but the original plan to stop going to Galveston for surgeries was eventually changed. For whatever reason or perhaps combination of factors, I was going back to Galveston. I believed back then, it might have been because the Chicago Hospital staff didn't feel it was able to properly handle my surgical needs. But then again, that's just a theory. Nevertheless, I was headed back to Galveston later that spring, and eventually, I stopped going to the Chicago Shriners Clinic altogether. One good piece of news came from my dermatologist sometime that spring who said my skin problem was a reaction to something. I don't remember what that "something" was, but he prescribed a medicated lotion with an annoying smell, which also stung when rubbed on. Then Eucerin lotion was rubbed in over the top of that for the dryness. Gradually over the months, my skin got better, and the severe face redness was pretty much gone by the end of my eighth-grade school year. I also ended using Eucerin lotion on my face every day even after the skin problem had cleared up. It made a huge difference in dryness and with how my skin actually felt. Now if I go without it, my facial skin feels tight, as if it's being stretched out, which is rather uncomfortable.

Chapter 21

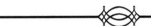

I think it was around March when my counselors Scott Vaughn, Mike Herbert, and a few of the other guys wanted to take Joey and me to a monster truck show, but instead of them driving down to us, it was Vicki and Diane who drove us up there. Kyle also decided to come along while everyone else stayed home. The entire drive up there, I was excited to see the guys and have a chance to hang out again. We first headed to Mike Herbert's apartment, and once we arrived nearby, Joey and I kept insisting we were at the right place, and we were both eager to see him. Mike wasn't home yet, so instead, we went to get some fried chicken nearby, and I honestly don't remember why, but Diane pulled me aside and lectured me about behaving poorly. I don't remember what I might have done to warrant the lecture, but at the time, she seemed to think I acted that way when I was around Joey, and my excitement to see the guys might have been misread. We went to a hotel nearby the same arena in Rosemont, and before Joey and I left with the guys, Kyle asked if he could join us. Kyle had actually gone to one with me the year before in Peoria when Bob took us, and it's something he was interested in. Anyway, they let him come, but that was when Joey saw Kyle's... let's just call it "jerk" side. Some may call it mean, rude, or whatever, but as we got out of the van, Joey was ready to push my wheelchair, but Kyle shoved him out of the way. They had a small shoving contest right there until one of the guys told Kyle to let Joey push my chair. I remember Joey later said that night, "I can't believe he wouldn't let me push my own brother." I agreed with Joey; after all, he is my brother and we only shared so much time together back then. The next morning, we all had lunch at the hotel with Mike before we went home, and that was the only time Diane ever met anyone from camp except at my graduation. I sometimes wish she could have come up for visitors' day at camp, but she was a busy lady, I guess.

Not too long after the trip to Chicago, I headed back to Galveston. But just a few days before I left, we switched my home health provider from Western Illinois Home Health Care to Spoon River Home Health. The majority of the WIHC nurses were older, and the Spoon River office was also closer, thus making it easier for them. I was introduced to two new nurses, Julie Sloan and Janet Scovil. I never enjoyed new nurses being trained, but the new home health was better all around. In a successful attempt to get on my good side, they both asked if there was anything they could get me while I was in Galveston, and it would be waiting till I got back. I was still into *Jurassic Park*, so I told them the Ford Explorer toy from the movie would be cool. It was a simple enough request, and they seemed happy to oblige. Some kids outgrow toys and childish things sooner than others. I always believed I was slower to move on from them because I didn't have much when I was younger, so it was in essence like I was making up for what I didn't have before. But either way, an offer to buy me something was always an effective way to get friendly with me back then. I know it was sometime during the spring, and I can't pinpoint exactly when, but it was around that time I estimate when my siblings were finally placed into foster care. My mom had been struggling for months, both financially and trying to mend things with Kirk or move on. Cassandra and Elizabeth started out in a home near Lake Bracken, while Joey and Elric shuffled among a few homes in Galesburg. One set of foster parents they had ate out for every meal and never cooked at home, while yet another had bars covering the windows. I hated the idea of those bars because I knew they could be a death trap in a fire. Finally, they ended up with Christine and Joe Spence in Galesburg. Ironically, I first became aware they were living there when I heard from Christine's sister-in-law Julie Bent, who was also a nurse of mine at Methodist, of an incident involving Joey and sugar all over the kitchen table.

On my flight to Galveston, I couldn't help but think to myself, *Here I go again.* I had assumed my previous stay had been my last surgery in Galveston, but it simply wasn't meant to be. And now this time, Merilyn was no longer there since she moved to Seattle. There were a few changes that year along with Merilyn being gone. Obviously, I had a new physical therapist, but I was also in a different room this time, and my surgery were two new procedures for me since my bedridden days back in 1990. My cheeks were somewhat tight, and it pulled my lower eyelids down, thus somewhat exposing the lower eye socket. It also kept my eyes from shutting tightly while sleeping, but so far, that wasn't a problem. The other surgery was lifting up my lower lip so it simply didn't hang so low or look so big. I didn't know what to expect from either surgery, but the lip surgery meant an entire week without solid food. And because removing the bandage was difficult, it meant I would be asleep for that too. Despite the longing torture for solid food, out of all my surgeries, I think that time was my easiest. All the other aspects during that particular stay simply made it less stressful. On the morning I was scheduled for surgery, the surgeons were running a little behind, which wasn't unusual. I was told it might be awhile, so I started watching *Return of the Jedi* until they came for me. My interest in *Star Wars* was obviously still growing. During the epic space battle near the end of the movie, it was finally time to go. Aww, man, you couldn't let me finish the movie? But I was told I could finish it later. When they are ready, they're ready. So Vicki said she would see me in a few hours, and I left on the gurney down to the surgical elevators, then down to the surgical rooms on the second floor. Those halls were colored annoyingly bright with sky blue and clouds painted on the walls. And then in the operating room, there were those creepy surgical lights with the pointed tip in the center. Those lights never changed much since the early days, and yet they creeped me out just the same every time. Thankfully, I was put to sleep just as easy as last time with minimal pain, and hours later, I awoke in the recovery room, where I dealt with the usual recovery room banter. "Can you cough for me?" "How are you doing?" "Ready to head back yet?" "We'll be going to your room soon." "Are you warm enough?" It could be worse, I guess. Vicki was waiting in my room when I got back, and I was always glad to have her there at those times. That was always when I was at my most helpless. I couldn't see anything, nor could I do anything for myself, because I didn't have my prosthesis on. So I was always thankful for her when I needed it most. Because all the surgery was on my face, it made it easier for me to be up and mobile in my wheelchair sooner. I was still tired though because the surgery and the healing always took a huge toll on my body. Vicki went back home for a few days because I was in my chair and would be all right by myself now that I wasn't stuck in bed. I had my Micro Machines, my Bon Jovi music, and even a remote for the TV this time. To my surprise, I even received a small care package from my school therapists at Lindbergh, which contained a few *Ghost Rider* comics, a Guns N' Roses CD, and some candy. It helped to know they were thinking of me and was always nice to have that distraction. Even though it seemed easier than other surgeries, my lip bandaged up slowly drove me crazy. I don't know how I lasted all those months back in 1990 without solid food and rarely a drop to drink. At least this time, I could still enjoy a liquid diet, but every food commercial I saw on TV that week was torture. The desire and cravings were almost constant.

The bandages below my eyes ended up falling off on their own just a day or two before they were to be removed. I was worried it was a bad thing that they fell off early, but it actually was just fine. Then came the day the doctor was to remove the bandaging from my lip. I was nervous beforehand, but I was already asleep when I was given something for the pain, and when I woke up, the bandaging was removed. I had to ask the nurse if they took it off already because I didn't feel a thing, and thankfully, the answer meant I could finally enjoy solid food again.

During the course of that week with the bandaging and its subsequent removal, the music therapist from the playroom was continuously working on a project with me. This project was another reason I was able to remain more positive during that particular stay. Using a video camera, she recorded me lip-synching Bon Jovi's "Living on a Prayer" at various locations throughout the hospital. We also made a banner we put up in my room with various positive quotes. Most of them were titles and lyrics of Bon Jovi songs, like "Keep the Faith" and "Living on a Prayer." While editing the video, I thought it would be a cool idea to cut into the real Bon Jovi music video during the guitar solo portion of the song and end it that way. When it was finished, we showed the nursing staff the video, and after seeing Jon Bon Jovi fly over the stage using a wire suspension, I think it was Bonnie Bishop who said, "I hope you never do that." The hardest part of those surgeries was going without food. Almost immediately after the bandaging on my lip was removed, I noticed a huge difference. Not only did my lip appear smaller, but I could now comfortably keep my mouth closed without effort. Prior to the surgery, my mouth usually hung open with a small gap. But the surgery came with a price because it required me to wear a chin strap for six months to support my lip and keep it from pulling down again. The chin strap itself was temporary until my face mask was finished. The mask was needed to support both my eyes and lips with the same device. But at least it was a newer clear plastic face mask this time. Everything about that mask was an improvement over the silicon mask years before. It was easier to put on, less hot, more comfortable, and didn't hinder my vision as much as the old face mask. Before I knew it, I was already back home in Rapatee. All my surgical stays in Galveston were about a month-long each time, but that stay seemed to go faster than the previous stays. Unfortunately, the following year wouldn't be so easy.

As always, I was glad to be back home, and this time, a surprise awaited me when I arrived. My new nurses kept their promise about buying what I asked for, but also to my surprise, Vicki decided to swap the bedrooms around again while I was gone. Gregg and David swapped with Mystic, and Jessica switched rooms with me. So Mystic and Jessica now shared the porch bedroom I had when I left, and I then had Jessica's old room to myself. Finally, I had the privacy I deserved and no longer trekked through three rooms to take a shower every day. The bathroom was connected directly to my bedroom, which made things way easier for my nurses and me. I could now be carried directly from my bed to the shower instead of transferring to the wheelchair and going back and forth. Jessica and Mystic, on the other hand, didn't get along so well most of the time. For the next few months, they always seemed to be at each other's throats, usually with Mystic being the drama queen and the one to overreact every time. One day that spring, I got a phone call from a lady who worked for the Starlight Foundation in Chicago. I asked Vicki her name, but she doesn't remember, and with so many people over the years, it's impossible. As a matter of fact, Vicki mixed up what I asked from Starlight Foundation with the Dream Factory, and I guess she forgot about my original DF wish entirely. Somebody told them all about me, and they decided to grant me a wish or two. The Starlight Foundation provided much the same thing as the Dream Factory in Pekin, only on a bigger scale you might say. I was told I could have two wishes, and I was given examples of what I might wish for. I could meet a famous actor or singer or even go on a trip. My first request was a no-brainer. I wished to meet Bon Jovi. She told me she would do her best and see what she could do. Secondly, after thinking about it, I thought it would be cool for the family to go on a vacation to Hollywood. But the catch was I wanted to go on a train so we could enjoy the scenery on the way there. I thought Hollywood would be cool because that's where the movie magic was made, TV shows were recorded, and it was the place most actors and movie stars themselves called home. I had hoped for a chance to be part of an audience of one of my favorite shows like *Full House, America's Funniest Home Videos*, or even *The Price Is Right*. But a trip to California wasn't meant to be, I guess, at least not yet. I don't remember what made me change my mind. I think it might have been the description and details of way more perks and potential excitement, but I decided on a trip to Orlando, Florida, and Disney World!

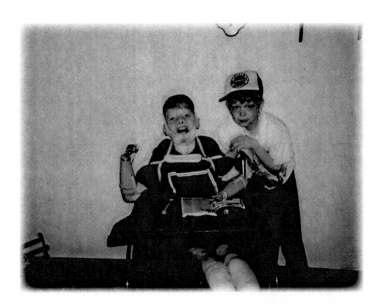

Chapter 22

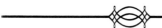

School at Lindbergh that spring seemed to be more difficult than usual. I had to wear my chin strap at school, and initially, I got a lot of questions about it and even more questions a month later when I changed to the face mask, but those were trivial problems compared to the other issues I faced almost daily. As they had the year before, my grandma and grandpa came to Lindbergh for Grandparents Day. But I noticed that very few of the eighth graders' grandparents came. I shrugged off, thinking I was too old for it, and was simply grateful they were still with me. I remember how I felt left out during Grandparents Day way back in second grade in Annawan. We were all asked to write a little description about our grandparents and put it on the blackboard for them to read and guess at. On mine, it read we always enjoyed popcorn and a movie every time we visited, but I hated being left out like that. At school, one way or another, it always seemed like I felt left out of something. Another early example of that would be the Boy Scouts. I remember during kindergarten or first grade, I went to an evening presentation at Galva Elementary about becoming a Boy Scout. Victor was a Boy Scout when he was younger, so naturally, I wanted to try it too, but for whatever reason, it never came to be. I also had a teacher that year that seemed somewhat rough around the edges. I've had way worse, but I don't know why she seemed to come across so grouchy and perhaps stern. During class, after finishing any work and assigned reading, I assumed I was free to read whatever book I currently had from the library. I would open the book and begin reading when she snapped it shut as if I did something wrong. I'd say I was finished with my work or whatever and, for reasons unknown, still wouldn't be allowed to read. Even if I sat idly for a few minutes, thinking enough time had passed, she would still snap my book shut with a glare. It wasn't just me she did that to, on more than one occasion I watched as she snapped shut the book of a classmate. I felt when she did that it kind of gave a mixed message. This is a school, right? Isn't reading in school during free time a good thing? Then there was everyday stress from a few of my classmates. Increasingly, I felt like I was on unequal and less friendly terms with some of them. To put it bluntly, I was smarter than most of them, but too often, I felt like they treated me opposite, and it seemed to me some thought they could boss me around like a younger child. One day, I brought my baseball card collection to show a few "friends" I regularly shared lunch with. That was a bad idea after one of them took a handful of them without asking. When I told him to give them back, he blew me off and walked away. I told one of my closer friends about it, but I never did get those cards back. Seriously, what kind of loser steals baseball cards or even anything from a disabled student? Especially when that student is fully aware of what was done. Later in the year, that same friend yelled at me for something innocent I said about him and his girlfriend. I actually was happy for him and meant no ill will, but he jumped down my throat, and that's when I realized he wasn't much of a friend anymore. He was focused on his girlfriend now, and I increasingly felt isolated, frustrated, and thinking perhaps I needed a change.

I came home a lot that spring, feeling disrespected and sometimes hurt. I no longer felt the connection with some of my classmates that I used to have. A few of those days, I called Diane and asked if I could stay the weekend or go out for dinner. Sometimes the answer was yes, but when I needed it, sometimes the answer was no. I don't think anyone truly knew the extent of my frustrations at the time. Whether it was my morning shower routine, school problems, or the usual staring in public, I felt sometimes like nobody could really relate to the various things I dealt with. I would go out into the grassy field near our house to be alone, or if need be, I'd ask if I could go to the stop sign past the north edge of town by myself. I could do so easily because there was a path next to the fence large enough for a vehicle, which kept me off the road. I needed to be alone with my emotions to let it out sometimes, and going for a stroll helped get my mind off things. Sometimes a person needs a place to get away from "it all," and for the most part, it helped. But one occasion as I was on my walk alone, some guy in a truck drove by slowly, and as he stared at me directly in the eye, he flipped me off. The whole purpose I went out there by myself was to momentarily leave it all behind, but even out there alone, my troubles still seemed to follow me There I was already struggling with aspects of my life when some asshole I never did anything to saw fit to make my life feel worse than it already was. Why does anyone feel the need to attack a person in such a way? It wasn't teasing or harassment; it was an attack. Because an attack meant ill will with the intention of harm. Did his own life suck so bad that he felt an attempt to ruin my day might brighten his own? What did I do to him other than be on the side of the road trying to forget the very same kind of thing I saw in his truck that day—human ugliness at its worst as I struggled with teenage stress, negative emotions, and so many other things the average normal teenager never dealt with.

Near the end of the school year was the annual Lindbergh School Olympics. It was basically our school challenging students from another in basic physical competitions like running and throw- ing. But obviously, some of the challenges were adapted to suit the limitations of the students with physical disabilities like myself. The competition was a welcome change of pace from the usual class schedule, and at the end of the school year was also the eighth grade end of year field trip. Because we were going to St. Louis, we actually had to be at school very early so our charter bus could leave on time. Unfortunately, because it was a charter bus, I couldn't bring my power chair. I hated being pushed around, but the only other option was to stay home. I brought along my headphones to listen to Bon Jovi, and our first stop was the St. Louis Science Center. This time, my visit was longer, and we were able to see more of the museum, including my first IMAX theater experience. The short definition of an IMAX theater is that it consisted of a *huge* screen with stunning realism. I was seated halfway down in an area for wheelchairs, but the room was still huge. When the film started, I immediately noticed my fear of heights began to show its ugly head. I was not expecting it at all, but the size of the theater combined with how high I was and the view of a helicopter flying over huge areas made it all too realistic. I was firmly on the ground in no danger, yet the view was telling my visual senses otherwise. I felt like I was going to fall or freak out, and I actually had to force myself to calm down by reminding myself I was perfectly safe where I was. At the gift shop that day was when I bought the first piece of my wolf figurine collection. I didn't really know what else to choose; I liked wolves, so I bought one, and I figured, why not start collecting them? Our second stop was the St. Louis Magic House. Back then, I had no idea what magic had to with learning and why it warranted a field trip visit. But when we arrived, I quickly realized the name was simply a clever way to get kids interested. The place was awesome with tons of hands-on learning, creativity, and problem-solving skills. I remember two rooms in particular at the magic house. The slanted room, which was basically a room inclined at an angle to make it appear as if standing at an angle even though you are actually standing straight up. The other was the room with the Tesla coil. It was a steel sphere with a slight electric current, and whenever a person touched it, their hair stood up on end without any danger of shock. At both museums, there were tons of exhibits, and it was a long day, so I don't remember a lot of them, but our final stop of the day was the St. Louis Union Station. At the time, I didn't realize it used to be a huge train station bustling with thousands of passengers every day. The original architecture still stands, but now, much of it is a mall filled with shops and restaurants. The first shop I went into was a shop for model train enthusiasts. Had I known earlier, I would have saved my spending money till then. I had wanted to get back into my train interest for years, and that shop only increased my desire. Not only did I wish I had more spending money, but I hated being pushed around when there was so much to see. Before we left, I did buy a new copy of Bon Jovi's *Young Guns II* soundtrack to replace the one Cassandra's friend "borrowed" back in Monmouth. And there was a decent selection of dining options at Union Station, including Hooters, but our group ended up choosing McDonald's. To be honest, back then, I thought Hooters was just a name. Had I known the facts, I might have tried to get Mr. Simpson to go there instead of McDonald's. I didn't complain back then though, because my taste in food was much different than it is now. Since that day, I have always wanted to return with spending money and see what I missed on my first visit, but I have yet to go back.

I don't recall exactly when it was that I decided which high school I was going to attend that fall. I considered all the pros and cons of both schools, including distance, school size, and the fact that as of late there were aspects of Lindbergh that had been bothering me that semester. After weighing my options, I changed my initial decision and chose to attend Spoon River Valley High School. Before the end of my final year at Lindbergh, my therapists and Lindbergh staff invited physical therapists who worked with another physically disabled student at Spoon River Valley. It was all the same stuff being shown to them as was when I first arrived at Lindbergh. Demonstrating and showing my new therapists the proper therapy techniques and other details involving my physical needs, limitations, and care. And then finally came eighth-grade graduation. For me, it felt like recognition of many accomplishments. Despite losing ground while hospitalized, I wasn't held back to make up for time missed. I faced obstacles and still managed to overcome them. During graduation, I was given an award for my reading accomplishments even though I was just barely outside the top 10 percent that year, not to mention my eighth-grade fall semester was my first and only time on the honor roll. My foster family was there, as well as the Wells and my grandparents. I remember wishing my mom could have seen my accomplishment, but she was still going through rough times. The entire occasion felt like a time of recognition and included a sense that we were all moving on to the next step in our lives. We were all going to new schools with new teachers where we would be the rookies in that part of life. Even our principal had decided it was time to retire and move on. After the graduation ceremony, I gave my Looney Tunes tie to Mr. Simpson as a kind of good-bye gift, and that was the end of my days at Charles A. Lindbergh Middle School.

Chapter 23

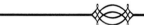

Yay, it was summertime again. Free from the chains of never-ending imprisonment known as school. I had a lot to look forward to that summer, and at the top of that list was our trip to Florida. With summer also comes inevitable water fights, but water didn't bode well when mixed with my first power chair. As it had the previous summer, I felt left out whenever there was a water fight with the neighbors and ended up joining in. The end result was usually my wheelchair failing on me and thus out of commission for a few weeks. I don't remember exactly how many times my chair broke down, but it was more than once. Then during the winter months, it was a different mobility problem when the slightest bit of snow would get caught on my belt drive. The snow would wedge between the belt and the rotor and make it come off or snap the belt in half. All four tires on that wheelchair were inflated, so flat tires tended to happen every now and then, especially in high school, when it seemed I was constantly running over thumbtacks. So that first wheelchair almost seemed to be out of service more than I actually used it. Originally, I wanted to take the train for our trip to Florida, but I was easily convinced to choose flying because getting down there faster meant we could stay longer. Jessica was afraid to fly and told me she would not go unless we took the train. I figured she would most likely change her mind by then, but due to recent conflicts at home, some with Mystic and whatever else, she moved out before our trip. Gregg and David were increasingly spending the night with their mom in preparation for finally moving back home with her later in the summer before school started again. I honestly wasn't looking forward to them leaving when the time came. Those boys were like little brothers, and they gave me somebody to hang out and do stuff with. One weekend, Kyle and I spent the night at the Wells'. We were there so we could go see *Lion King* the next day with Diane. If you ask me, I don't think anyone can ever be too old or too young for any Disney movie. A guy like Kyle proves that theory. Despite his quite occasional temper and attitude, even he liked Disney movies for the most part. Heck, even years later, he watched *The Little Mermaid* with me one night on the Disney Channel after not seeing it for a few years. Before we saw it, I had read a review that said the *Lion King* was a modern-day remake of *Bambi*. Even Diane's neighbor kid warned us it was sad as we left the house to go see it. As anyone whose seen the *Lion King* knows, yeah Simba witnessing the death of his father was indeed sad, but the movie was excellent and still remains my favorite Disney film of all time. I loved the music so much that I eventually bought the soundtrack. Obviously, I wasn't the only one to think the music was great because it became the biggest-selling soundtrack for an animated film, and I watched when it won Academy Awards for best original score and best original song. The movie itself resonated within me the troubles I faced in my own life. As the character Rafiki said, "Yes, the past can hurt, but the way I see it you can either run from it… or learn from it." At the end of the movie, after all his pain and personal struggle, Simba climbed atop Pride Rock to take his rightful place. His ascension was symbolic and inspiring to me because despite the difficulties, he overcame them in the end.

Finally, sometime around June or July, we left for Florida. Diane would keep an eye on Max for me, and I promised to bring a gift back for her and Bob. We headed up to Chicago and stayed at a hotel not far from Midway Airport because our flight was the next morning. I remember Gregg and David acting up before we left, and Vicki threatened to leave them behind and bring along Joey and Elric instead. The next morning, we were up early so I could shower, and then of course, there was my usual boring morning care. Then we had a quick breakfast and went to the airport. After the van was parked in the lot, we rode a shuttle to the terminal, and after taking care of our luggage and tickets, we met up with the lady from the Starlight Foundation. She had balloons for me, and in my opinion, she seemed somewhat surprised by my appearance. A person being shocked by my appearance is nothing new and will always be a possibility. I occasionally chat online with somebody I've never met in person, and I just can't convey how extreme my burns really are. Until they meet me in person, my descriptions of myself can only do so much, and meeting me in person can be an eye-opener for many people. Anyhow, we talked for a bit and thanked her for all she had done. It wasn't easy to fulfill the wish because supposedly a former volunteer/employee of the foundation had stolen funds meant for granting wishes. Whether it actually happened or not, I don't know, but if it did, they should be truly ashamed, and I believe karma will hit with the force of a ton of bricks. Over the years, I flew a lot, and for one reason or another, there tended to be occasional delays. That day was no exception as the flight was delayed hour by hour due to mechanical issues. It wasn't planned, but we actually had lunch/dinner before we finally boarded in mid/late afternoon. That flight was my first nonhospital flight. For once, I could enjoy the flight without the stress and worry of knowing the destination was a hospital. That time, the destination was a fun, magical, and awesome place totally opposite from a hospital. But about halfway into the flight, I realized I should have stayed away from the soda I had prior to the flight. I was holding it for a while, but I realized I wasn't going to be able to make it until we landed in Orlando. I told Vicki of my "predicament" as she sighed and wondered what to do. I couldn't just sit there, and my need for relief was sucking the fun out of the flight. So despite all the unwanted attention and curious eyes, Vicki carried me to the lavatory, where she helped me deal with my business. Once back at my seat, I enjoyed that "ahhh, much better" feeling until we landed in Orlando around 8:00 p.m. or so. Our arrival day was somewhat a shame. Because of arriving so late, the sun had already gone down before we left Orlando Airport. We were greeted by a representative from the Give Kids the World Village who drove us there in the van we would be using all week.

Quoted directly from their website, "Give Kids the World is a nonprofit organization that exists only to fulfill the wishes of all children with life-threatening illnesses and their families from around the world to experience a memorable, joyful, cost-free visit to the Central Florida attractions, and to enjoy the magic of Give Kids the World Village for as long as there is a need." GKTW really is a village; it's not a metaphor for their organization. Every family stayed in individual villas, and I was amazed at how far they went to make families feel truly at home. It in fact was a home because it had all the amenities, including TVs, furniture, kitchen, bedrooms, bathrooms, and anything else you could think of. Aside from the family villas, there was the main office, where we signed in, and we learned what was planned and/or available for us throughout the week. Then there was the Gingerbread House restaurant, where every meal was served by Perkins, and nearby that was the ice cream parlor Caboose. But we spent most of our short-lived free time at the Castle of Miracles. Outside it was a small stream full of loose change and a carousel. Inside were a gaming room and other rooms such as the main throne room. In the throne room, there were golden glass stars with the names of all the former wish kids, which now included mine. Last but not least was the pool, complete with wheelchair ramp and the nearby fishing pond as well. The village had so many fine details like Ol' Elmer, the talking tree, and even the village cat. When I looked up the official website, I saw how much has been added since I visited all those years ago. Not only is there even more to see and do, but there's even more rooms with more golden stars representing all the former wish kids. If allowed, I'd pay to for a chance to stay there again even without all the generosity I was shown during my original stay, if only to revisit those memories I made the first time.

After we were up and ready early the next morning, we had breakfast and then went to the main office to see about our itinerary and options for our week. From there, we went to Magic Kingdom for our first park of the week. We did so much throughout the week among four different parks I can't be absolutely certain what order we visited them in. But I know Magic Kingdom was first, and as a matter of fact, it was the only park we went to twice. We rode the monorail from our parking spot up to the gate area, and the excitement was rising. You can't help but feel the childlike magic when you visit Disney World, which explains why so many adults love it as much as kids do. Just past the gate was the Walt Disney World Railroad, but what really caught my attention was Cinderella's castle, which loomed not far in the distance past Main Street, U.S.A. I was excited to finally find out just what was inside the castle, and not to mention visit the spots where my then-favorite show *Full House* filmed scenes the year before. Inside the castle wasn't what I expected, but it was awesome nonetheless. It had a shop inside with cuckoo clocks, miniature castles, swords, etc. I had saved up my money prior to the trip, and that's where I found what I wanted. I liked crystal collectibles, but what I wanted was a bit pricey, considering how small it was. It was still early, and I didn't want to blow all my cash that early in one place, so I waited till later on. I rode as many things as I could safely, but I still regret missing out on a few rides. Every ride I did I rode more than once before the week was over. Some of my favorite rides were Peter Pan's Flights, the Haunted Mansion, the Mad Tea Party, and last but not least, Pirates of the Caribbean. Some of the kids split up to attack the park on their own and ride what I wouldn't or couldn't, for example Thunder Mountain Railroad and Space Mountain. I would have rode Space Mountain, but I wasn't confident I could safely ride it. When Joey rode it during his trip in 2012, I asked him about it, and he said I probably would have flown out because of individual seats, so I obviously made the right choice. I loved spinning around endlessly on the Mad Tea Party ride, but Vicki and especially Mystic sure didn't. As a matter of fact, all week long, Mystic missed out on rides even I was willing to ride. Some of them made sense, but others it was plain silly she skipped on. Magic Kingdom was special because it represented the magic you always saw on TV but always seemed so far and out of reach. It was always that place I never got to go while the lucky people did, but now it was my turn. I was finally at the wonderful place I'd seen so many times and the ultimate destination of so many young and young at heart. One of the most special moments for me at the Magic Kingdom was actually a fairly simple one. On our way through the park, we came across Cinderella, who kindly talked with me and politely asked questions I was happy to answer. Some people when asking questions can be too nosey, impolite by talking to those with me instead of directly to me, or condescending by talking to me as if I was much younger. But she talked with me on an equal level, respectful of my age and intellect. Before we parted, I had my picture taken, and then she asked if she could give me a kiss on my cheek. I gladly said yes, and I'll never forget that magical moment when she looked past my scars and saw what was inside; it always makes me smile when I think about it.

I don't remember which park we went the next day, but it was either Universal or MGM Studios. The only thing that mattered really was that we had fun, so I'll describe our visit to Universal first. Universal had more rides suited for older riders unlike Magic Kingdom, where it's all fantasy focused mostly on family and children. The first thing we did was go inside the actual studio. Nothing was being filmed at that time, but the group tour was set up like an audience, and we participated in a mock game show. This gave it the feeling of being like an actual game show. We didn't see any stage performances at Magic Kingdom but after the studio "show," we saw the

Ghostbusters live show. That one was actually pretty cool with decent effects. The actors were either in front of or behind a screen, which made it appear as if the ghosts or monsters were right there in front of them. The rest of our day was all rides, and they had some cool ones. But Mystic opted out of almost all of them, her loss. There was the King Kong ride, where we rode an elevated tram above the city streets, the Earthquake ride, Jaws, E.T. Adventure, and the Back to the Future ride. Those are the main rides I remember because to me they were the most fun. The earthquake and Jaws ride both had flame elements, which didn't actually bother me, but it was a good scare, although I could feel enough heat from the flame, which did trigger old memories. The E.T. Adventure ride was similar in setup to Peter Pan's ride, but instead of flying on a pirate ship over London and Neverland, you ride a bicycle flying through the forest. Back to the Future was actually more than I expected. I got in the DeLorean, and I assumed a small screen was right in front; I was wrong. The car moves forward into a room with other DeLoreans and a huge screen. It was almost identical to the OMNIMAX screen I saw in St. Louis, and combined with the 3-D realism of the footage, it made my fear of heights kick in when I didn't want it to. I honestly enjoyed the ride, but it seemed intense, and Vicki even teased me for losing my hat. Earlier that day was one of my favorite souvenir picture memories of our trip. There was a photo op for $15, where you could get a professional photo taken next to a life-size *T. rex* and jungle explorer from *Jurassic Park*. I couldn't pass up the opportunity and eagerly had my photo taken with Kyle, Mystic, Gregg, and David. It was a fun memory and cool to see the *T. rex* up close, but Gregg and David never smiled much for photos. At all the parks, I had special privileges like line skipping, which was required for disabled guests, but I also had a golden star pinned to my hat to show I was a Wish kid. At Universal Studios, my star meant a free dinner for the entire family at Hard Rock Cafe Orlando at Universal Studios. Our server was an awesome guy who went above and beyond the duty of a server to make our visit a great time. I was told I could have whatever I wanted and immediately decided on a juicy T-bone steak. That was my first time at a Hard Rock, and visits years later to one in Indianapolis were nothing like my first experience in Orlando. Of course, Orlando was high traffic in terms of customers, but the place was like one big party while we were there. Servers were dancing around even on tables, and the entire time, I was wondering if it was an everyday thing. My steak was succulent, and honestly safe to say, it was my best and favorite meal that entire week.

Disney's MGM Studios seemed bigger than Universal even though the latter had more rides we actually went on. My favorite ride by far at MGM and probably the whole week was Star Tours. The area around the entrance was decorated to look like a scene on Endor from *Return of the Jedi* with crashed speeder bikes and a not-quite-life-size Imperial Walker standing ominously over the pathway. The ride itself was awesome, and afterward, I remember thinking about how they achieved the sensation of our ship jumping into hyperspace. My only regret was not buying anything from the *Star Wars* gift shop just after the ride. The *Star Wars* fan inside me was still growing, and even though I didn't buy anything, the ride was probably a big influence on further boosting my interest. Most of the things we did at MGM were actually shows. We saw the Indiana Jones stunt spectacular but missed part of that one because we were late. Then we saw Muppet*Vision 3D, which was the only non-live performance show other than part of the behind-the-scenes studio tour. We saw *The Little Mermaid* live show, and like everything Disney, I love how they go all out to make the experience authentic and magical. It was in a room made to feel like an underwater cavern, with bubbles and misting. The room itself was nice and cool, which made it all that much better cause, it provided a chance to get out of the Florida heat. The heat and daily thunderstorms were probably the biggest issues we had during our stay. The storms slowed us down, but they at least helped keep the heat from being overly oppressive all day long. My favorite live show during our trip was also at MGM, and that was the *Beauty and the Beast* stage show. The show only lasted about a half hour, but it seemed to cover everything shown in the movie. Everything, including the costumes, acting, singing, and sets, matched the movie perfectly. I will always believe Disney can be enjoyed by everyone kids, adults, even men. I know for a fact this is true. Anyhow, the reason Beauty and the Beast is my favorite princess/fairy tale type animated film is that despite Beast's/ Prince Adam's fearsome, scary, animalistic, unhuman appearance, that Belle could still see something inside. Occasionally I fantasize of getting my unburned body back in the same way Beast does. Floating up into a cradle of blinding light and then settling back down as an able bodied person again. And I bet many disabled people often imagine the same or similar fantasy. During the show, I remember eating my first foot-long hotdog. It might seem like a small detail, but it was my first time eating a foot-long. Combined with the show and the quality of the hot dog, I compare it to the traditional hot dog at a baseball game. I don't remember if they were all part of one studio tour or split into two, but one of my favorite parts was the actual behind-the-scenes studio tour. For easier reading, I'll just describe it all as it happened as one, albeit long tour. The first part was a movie set demonstrating how they shot water scenes with miniatures, blue screens, and special effects like fans and blowing water to simulate a hurricane at sea. Next I think was actually inside the working studio. The whole family got to see a real taping of a show called *That's My Dog* on what was then called the Family Channel. Then we saw the behind-the-scenes magic of how they created our favorite animation. It included a short film describing the process and a walk through the studio where you could see through the actual artists at work, and that was followed up by displays of concept art from recent films like *Lion King*, as well as my first glimpse of Pocahontas sketches. Still the tour wasn't over. After that, we boarded a tour tram which took us through the lots only accessed by the tour. In the "boneyard," we saw vehicles and set parts from old movies like Herbie and even the brain-shaped ship from *Flight of the Navigator*, which I particularly liked. The ride then proceeded to Catastrophe Canyon, which gave the riders the experience and feel of a real movie set. I had seen vacation video prior, so I had an idea of what to expect as the ground started to shake, boulders began to fall, followed by a tanker truck sliding down the mountainside as it leaked fuel, and of course, fireballs that I could feel the heat from until a waterfall came out of nowhere extinguishing the flame and ending the ride. From there, the tram simply took us back the way we came. For anyone who goes to MGM, aka Hollywood Studios, I highly suggest the studio tours. There was one ride I skipped out on at MGM, and that was the Tower of Terror. If I remember correctly, I think I opted to skip it because of my issue with heights. We did so much at MGM, I'm surprised we accomplished as much as we even did.

We had many parks to choose from during our stay, but the one we missed out on was Epcot. We had the chance to go, but I think we all decided on a second visit to Magic Kingdom so we could see the evening light parade. During that second visit, I rode all the same rides again except the Mad Tea Party. I still wanted to buy the crystal castle from the shop inside Cinderella's castle, but Vicki suggested that if I buy one of the more affordable but bigger castles, I could buy a new entertainment center for my TV when we got back home. So after thinking it over, I decided to get the affordable, albeit bigger one, and that was my biggest souvenir purchase that week. We saw the light parade late in the evening, and it was awesome. Every year in East Peoria, they hold the annual festival of lights parade and then display the floats afterward until the holidays are over. Those are cool in their own right, but the Disney parade was totally tricked out with synced music, and even the costumes themselves were lighted. That night on the ride back to the village, I was totally exhausted. The whole drive back, I just wanted to lean on something and sleep because we just couldn't get back to our villa fast enough. Even though it seemed like we were nonstop busy with visiting parks, we did have one night that week when parents went out and the kids stayed at the village. Vicki, Lee, and the other parents went out for dinner, and we stayed back and mostly played video games that night. When we went back to our villa, we were surprised to see plush *Lion King* Simbas waiting on the kitchen counter for all of us. Vicki said somebody must have brought them while we were gone but later admitted she and Lee bought them for us while during their night out. The week seemed to fly by so fast, even quicker than camp did. I did get something to bring back for Bob and Diane, and even though I don't recall exactly what it was, I do know it had something to do with Diane's pig collection.

On our last full day in Florida, we went to Sea World. That park was different because most of it was animal attractions and shows instead of rides. We didn't get to see as much as I would have liked because Vicki decided we should leave early so we could get packed in time for our flight back home the next morning. But luckily, we did get to see the main attraction, Shamu. Even though it wasn't the real original Shamu, basically all the shows were still known by that name. We were seated halfway up and just barely out of reach of the biggest splashes. Before the show started, kids would run away crying to their parents after being splashed. It was a fun show and by far the best live animal performance I've seen. To my surprise, after the show and most of if not all the crowd had left, I was invited down next to the tank by one of the trainers so I could see the orca up close. Seeing the whale up close and personal was a memorable experience. Those beautiful animals are so much bigger in person, and you realize they truly deserve our respect and protection so future generations may enjoy them. The trainer talked to us about the orcas, told us their names, and even did a few simple movement tricks. Then the trainer asked me, "Would you like to get wet?" I assumed the whale would jump out of the water and I'd be drenched by the wave and splash.

But instead, the trainer gave a hand signal and the orca dipped its mouth in the water and repeatedly sprayed water on me until I was thoroughly soaked. Afterward, my first thought was, *I can't believe I was spit on by a whale.* We then proceeded to the shark exhibit, but unfortunately for me, part of it was inaccessible to wheelchairs, which was disappointing. It wasn't long after that we decided to leave, but on our way out, Kyle bought a pearl oyster for $10 and the pearl inside was supposedly valued at $40. I still dream of going back to Florida one day to hopefully visit GKTW and revisit those memories from that magical week. Aside from burn camp, our trip to Florida is one of my favorite memories from those years and by far my favorite vacation experience. I got to see and do things I could only imagine. Until then, those things always seemed out of reach and meant for somebody else to enjoy. I found out many years later that the wishes granted to me were meant for chronically and terminally ill children. Those kids deserved it all much more than I do, I think. Because of what children like me and others go through, we miss out on things in life we otherwise wouldn't get to see and do. It's because of my burns that I definitely missed out on many things some people take for granted. And there will always be things I will miss out on as life continues. Generous people and organizations like the Starlight Foundation, Dream Factory, Give Kids the World, Shriners, and IFSA, which have helped me over the years make life easier by making it more enjoyable with experiences and opportunities I'd otherwise never have. I try my best every day to earn the generosity I was shown and give back any way I can because I truly am grateful for all that's been done for me over the years. I want to give to others as unfortunate as I was so that they too might experience that same joy and happiness.

After our Florida trip, I immediately looked forward to burn camp. I was excited to tell everyone at camp all about my trip. But in early August, the day had come for Gregg and David to move back home. I wasn't looking forward to them leaving for good and having nobody to do stuff with, but I was happy for them. Of course, they were obviously more excited to go home than anyone else. On the day we left Rapatee to drop them off at their mom's, they were so excited they didn't seem to care how much Vicki and I would miss them. The original plan was to drop them off after a good-bye lunch. But they were in such a rude hurry Vicki just dropped them off, then we went to lunch, and that was the end of it. Gregg and David gone on the weekends meant boring days, but now I had to adjust to them being gone altogether. By then, Joey and Elric had moved in with Christine and Joe Spence in Galesburg but hadn't yet spent the night at my house. After the excitement to Florida, summer itself seemed to pass me by until once again it was time for burn camp.

My third year at camp was my first year in unit 3. The age groups were separated into different cabin units. And unit 3 was the highest age group up to the graduation age of sixteen. I had two more years left at that point, and I was already wondering what I would do after I graduated and couldn't be a camper anymore. But later I eventually heard whispers that Kathy Haage, Dottie Ahbe, and others were possibly thinking of starting a new training program to allow former campers to become counselors. Supposedly, it was initially created to specifically allow me to return. My cabin that year was Blue Jay. The unit 2 cabins were named after trees, and in unit 3, they were birds. Most of if not all the same guys were back again, plus or minus one or two, but there were a few years when one of my counselors would be assigned to another cabin and perhaps the next year it was switched up. Those years made it slightly harder to find time to talk to whichever counselor wasn't assigned with me. Just hanging out and talking about my year and everything going on was always a great way to connect. Having somebody who took the time to be genuinely interested in what I had to say made me feel appreciated and accepted. There are so many years that seem to meld together that as time has passed I can't remember every tiny detail from every year at camp. But I think I can honestly say I have at least one good memory from every year. One particular memory from burn camp '94 was our cabin skit. All the cabins were performing skits in the lodge one evening during an all-camp activity. Our cabin had rehearsed prior, and when it was our turn, we all came out in front of everyone crudely dressed up as Oompa Loompas. A tape was played, and we stood there singing the song, squatting up and down like they did in the original movie version of *Willy Wonka & the Chocolate Factory.* I remember thinking we looked ridiculous and everyone was laughing, but camp was always the kind of place where extreme goofing off was accepted and normal. That actually wasn't the first time my cabin purposely embarrassed itself. The first year when the cabins exchanged volunteers for the fashion show, our cabin dressed up as girls. Some of us had on makeup, crude bikini bras, and yarn for girly blond hair. I honestly don't know which was funnier to everyone else, but we were all in it together, and it was all in good fun. That year was also the year we started the annual fun fair held on visitors' day. We still started off with the fire apparatus parade, followed by lunch and sponsor presentations. Then after the campers sang the thank-you song to the sponsors, we typically started the fair. Basically, it's more or less a carnival, minus the bulky mechanical rides. Things have switched up over the years to keep things fresh, but normally, we always have a bouncy house, slide, dunk tank, face painting, popcorn stand, snow cones, game booths with prizes, and last but not least, a good humor truck with a ton of ice cream. Since the fun fair tradition began that year, it has always been a highlight of the week, and while writing this, we've only had to cancel once due to bad weather. But quite a few, I've had to stay inside for a portion of the fun fair afternoon because of hot summer weather. It's just a fact of life as a burn survivor. It'll never change, so I deal with it the best I can. Also, if I remember correctly, that year I was fortunate enough to get a quick ride in one of the helicopters that landed at camp. During those first few years, we usually had visits from area medical helicopters. The campers were allowed to see them up close inside and out, but obviously, they couldn't give rides because the number of campers who would miss out would just be unfair. But that year, I was allowed a quick ride after the rest of camp went back to their individual cabins. As we did a circle around the area, I remember thinking two things. I was amazed at how smooth the flight was and also at how many lakes there were in the area. That ride was awesome, and to me, it was a substitute for all the things I couldn't do.

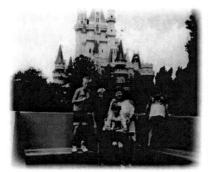
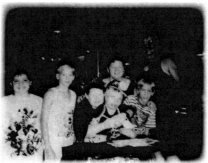

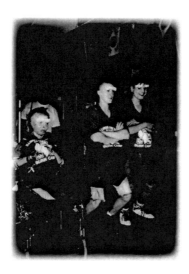

Chapter 24

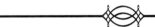

The next few months all the way until the end of the school year would be full of changes. Topping that list was my first year of high school. Just one week before school started, a few of my favorite faces from Galveston came up to prepare me and my new school for re-entry into a normal school setting. If I remember correctly, Catherine from child life and Patricia Blakeney were there to do so. I was excited to have them come see me in my home state for once instead of down in Galveston. Perhaps too excited because I was asked to say something on video for the entire school to see, and I honestly admit I didn't take it very seriously and my goofing off made a poor first impression. When my first day arrived, I was actually allowed to come in late while the school had an assembly in the gym to talk about a new student. Catherine and Pat talked about what happened to me and supposedly about all the details, like why I needed a wheelchair and my prosthetics, and answered any questions. I was picked up by P. J. Platt with his van because his son was also in a wheelchair. I arrived just as the assembly was nearing its end, and I was then asked to come into the gym. I was very hesitant, shy, and fearful of going out in front of everyone. All eyes would be on me, and I was not comfortable with that kind of attention whatsoever. But I went out, and all seemed quiet as I could see a few shocked faces and curious glances. They introduced me, I quietly waved hello, and that was pretty much it. Thankfully, that first day was a half day, which allowed me to slowly adjust to my new school without too much anxiety in one day. But first, I was introduced to my school aide Carl Sherman. He helped me with everything I needed in school. When he wasn't in the elementary building helping Travis Platt, he helped me with things like getting my books and stuff and getting to the next class, bringing my portable fan, lunch prep, and my more personal needs. The first day was focused mostly on getting my bearings and finding out what classes I'd have and where they would be. One advantage I immediately noticed was the A and B day schedule. The different days had their own set of classes, which at least made homework assignments easier to complete because it meant more time to complete them. The first disadvantage was the absence of my cousin Nick. Going to school with him was a big reason I chose Valley in the first place, so not having him there just sucked. He ended up going to Canton High School, where he stayed until graduating. I was also reintroduced to my new therapists, and Carl was shown how to do a few things in a private room set aside for my personal needs. That sums up the basics of my first two days of high school.

The other big change was mostly at home. After Gregg and David had moved out, Vicki then switched foster care providers from Catholic Social Services to Bridgeway. With so much that happened over the years, it's hard to remember the exact dates of some things, but I can usually estimate close enough to keep it all in order. I know it was sometime around the beginning of school/fall when the first two kids from Bridgeway moved in. Their names were Alisha and Eric. I actually didn't know it at the time, but recently, I found out from Vicki that Bridgeway allowed only two fosters because it was treatment care. Basically, treatment care is an alternative to being placed in an institutional setting and combines traditional foster care with elements of institutional care for kids with severe problems. To me, it didn't appear to be much of a difference, but after switching to Bridgeway, it seemed as if every kid had problems of some sort. Whether it was a lack of respect for rules and/or authority, drugs, running away, fighting, stealing, etc., there was always something. Eric was slightly older than Alisha, and in the beginning, most of the problems were from him. He mentioned early on he didn't care if he went to jail, but Vicki tried to instill fear in him by making him realize it was not where he wanted to end up. I truly believed Vicki was being honest when she said she didn't want to see him end up in jail. But as time went on, his behavior worsened as he fought with his sister and became increasingly combative. I don't recall exactly when, but eventually, the day came when he just did not care to listen to anyone at all. Vicki had him pinned on the floor, trying to get him to calm down and do as he was told, but he refused to listen and spewed obscenities left and right. When Eric got the chance, he was out the door and took off running down the road. Vicki was in no hurry to catch him because she figured on letting him walk away some energy while we got into the van to follow and bring him back. We followed him on his attempt to run away to Macomb, where supposedly his mom lived. He was defiant and continued to walk down the road. Vicki kept trying to make him change direction by making him second-guess his route. Eventually, Vicki had enough, and he got in the van, and we went back home. I don't remember how he left for good, whether he ran way, moved to a new home, or the police came for him. Around close to the same time they moved in, Vicki also got a Chihuahua puppy and named it Bailey. But unfortunately, also that fall my cockatiel Duncan passed away suddenly. I did get another cockatiel, which also died almost immediately while I was at school not long after we got it. I came home, and there was a blue parakeet sitting in the cage. Vicki and Diane tried to tell me it was the same bird as before, and honestly, I was insulted by the fact that they thought I was gullible or dumb enough to believe them.

Bob and Diane had big changes going on too. Supposedly somebody complained about how my staying with the Wells overnight sometimes was against the rules. According to DCFS, I wasn't allowed to stay overnight at an uncertified home without permission, which didn't really make sense because other than staying with the Wells, often I did stay overnight with my nurse Janet Scovill in Avon a few times as well. So in order for me to be able to stay overnight at the Wells, they had to become foster parents. From the very beginning, Diane told me that no matter what, I was always most important and that a new foster kid in their home wasn't going to change anything. I stayed the weekend with them when their first foster kid stayed as sort of a trial run. His name was Michael Frohm. He was about two years younger than me and had a variety of problems I won't go into details on. I was basically there to be a friend and make him feel welcome so that he might feel comfortable enough to move in with the Wells. That first weekend was pretty much the same as my first few days with Vicki. We went shopping, treated him to his favorite food, etc., all to make him feel at ease and welcome. When the weekend was over, he seemed ready to move in, and I went back home to Rapatee, where high school life was still fresh and new.

Kyle was still a grade behind me, and even though we were in the same building, I still felt somewhat alone. My first lunch at school was awkward because even though I was invited to a table by a few students, I was nervous as everyone watched me as I ate. I always hated that kind of attention, and I probably still would now, but I just wanted to eat my meal in peace without everybody watching my tiniest movement. Even though, I appreciated their efforts to be friendly, and if it were today, I probably would make a stronger effort to participate. I just can't change my shyness in crowds; it will always be a part of who I am. I don't want to be a loner, but my hearing, combined with my shyness, and larger crowds just made it uncomfortable for me at lunch. The next day, I admittedly sat on the other end of the cafeteria with a different crowd in an effort to avoid the stares and attention from the day before so I could simply eat my lunch in peace. As I settled in to high school life, I met Cozette Hoover, who was the elementary speech therapist. Even though I didn't need speech therapy, she took it upon herself to basically be a friend and was tasked with a few simple evaluation tests early on. But eventually, she started coming over for high school lunch period to just be friendly. Maybe it didn't seem like I appreciated her presence sometimes, but that was just my teenage rebellious side because often she asked me to talk during lunch and I refused. I actually did appreciate having her for lunch, but I simply didn't talk much while eating, and I still don't. Eventually, we had our own little "round table" at one end of the cafeteria. Early on that year, aside from any evaluations I might have been given by Mrs. Hoover, I was also given a few by Mrs. Walters. One of which was a test that evaluated my recognition of roadway signs. I never forgot when she told me I scored the average of a seventeen-year-old, and I was still just under fifteen.

Despite the effort by Mrs. Hoover and anyone else to make me feel more welcome, incidents with other students were inevitable. One of the first I remember early on in the year happened during my final class of the day, biology. Biology was one of those classes for me that proved I lagged behind in certain areas compared to the rest. Even though I thought it interesting enough, the number of details, terms, definitions, and even math made it difficult for me. But the incident involved Ryan A. passing me a note from a female student who I won't name. It mentioned how she had noticed me since the first day, blah, blah, blah, etc., and honestly it seemed to lack sincerity. I was hopeful it might indeed be genuine but didn't actually think it was. Ryan probably assumed I wasn't smart enough to realize it came from him when actually my first thought was that it was probably a cruel joke at my expense. I showed Vicki the note; she called his parents and thus confirmed my suspicions. It was a mean joke—though I wasn't surprised, to be honest—but at least it didn't involve the physical harassment I endured later on. In a few cases that first year, I admit some of those occasions I probably over-reacted to others around me. I perceived the slightest glare, stare, or mockery aimed at me in effort to tease or harass me, and I simply wouldn't accept the tiniest bit even if I had gotten it all wrong. So even though I had troubles for the most part, I dealt with it. Then there were my classes. Biology was probably the second toughest class my freshman year right after math. I despised math with a passion, and high school math further proved just how far I lagged behind in certain areas because of my time in the hospital. Even with the A and B days, it was still difficult, and I struggled increasingly as the year progressed. The classes that always seemed easiest to me were computer, business, and history classes. Prior to high school, I used computers a little bit at Lindbergh, but I hadn't taken any actual typing classes. When I first started, I was typing with one hook, but my teacher suggested I try with both, and over time, my speed and accuracy improved. At my fastest, I was typing up to 40 wpm aver-age when I used both hooks. That first year, I used Mrs. Fulton's room as my locker, homeroom, and study hall. Basically, I kept my books and things on a designated desk table and spent any free time between classes there finishing any assignments, reading, or therapy on the table, which was kept in her room at the time. I had to have my therapy somewhere, and at the time, it was the only place for it. My birthday that year fell on a school day, and the celebration was a fairly simple one that year. In my English class with Mr. Knox, who was also Vicki's stepbrother, he asked the class to sing "Happy Birthday." It's always nice to get a "Happy Birthday" even though it was too much attention. That evening at home, Vicki picked up a Bigfoot pizza from Pizza Hut, and other than Diane giving me my own copy of *Jurassic Park*, that was pretty much it. But it was enough just to have my own copy of *Jurassic Park*, because it had taken a year and half just to get it on video, compared to less than a half year wait from theater to DVD today. I saw a couple months before that it would be released on my birthday and begged Diane right then to reserve a copy for me. Obviously, she did, and I relived the excitement of seeing *Jurassic Park* for the first time on my own TV.

Chapter 25

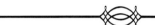

During those late months in 1994, Joey also started spending the night occasionally. If I had a rough week, I'd ask Vicki if he could stay, and then I'd call him up. Without Gregg and David around, more often than not, I was bored, unless I went to Diane's for the weekend or Lee's grandson Dustin spent a night or two. As I adjusted to high school and settled into a routine, I continued my lunches with Mrs. Hoover. We talked about random stuff, but one day in early December, I mentioned living with my aunt Leslie in Farmington for a short time back in the fall of 1988, and I had a girlfriend named Amanda. I couldn't remember her last name, but I told her how I had went by her old house, hoping to say hello, and was told she lived down the street but never did find her. I also told her she had a younger sister named Alicia. In respect to their privacy, I won't use their last names or go into heavy details. But I realized it was the same Amanda after Mrs. Hoover told me her last name and that she had been through a lot over the past two or three years. Mrs. Hoover then said she would get her phone number and we'd go from there. I don't remember who called who, but I was both nervous and excited when she called. I didn't really talk to anyone else on the phone, except for Joey and my grandparents every now and then, so talking to a girl on the phone was a new experience for me. As I said above, to protect their privacy I won't go into details, and there's no easy way to mention this, but it's still an important factor in our relationship. At just fourteen years old Amanda became pregnant, and her baby Zachary was born with cerebral palsy. She had been through a lot and, just like me, was forced to grow up too quick. After we set it all up, Vicki and I picked her and Zachary up at her house in Farmington. More than anything, I was very nervous, and it was awkwardly quiet in the van. We stopped to pick up Dustin and found out he had already met her because her grandparents lived next to his grandma. We slowly warmed up and talked a little bit, but that day was also the same day my grandparents were visiting to give me Christmas gifts. I introduced Amanda and said she was my girlfriend from back in '89, though technically it was late '88. In 1989, ironically, I spent more time with her younger sister Alicia because she was sent to Yates City for school and I'd chase and tease her during recess. Alicia used to tell me, "My sister hates you now," but I always just shrugged it off. Times sure changed for everyone. I remember being somewhat embarrassed by the gifts I asked for from Grandma. Yes, I got what I asked for, but opening gift wrapping with Yakko, Wakko, and Dot from *Animaniacs* in front of a "potential" girlfriend just felt un-macho so to speak. We watched TV and hung out in my room a bit, just chatting about stuff. All the while, Alisha loved watching Zachary while we did so. We then came out into the living room toward the end of her stay, and Amanda asked me to sit on the couch with her. Kyle even said I should sit with her, but I was conflicted. Part of me very much wanted to, but I was surprised by how fast sitting together happened, and the fact that my stomach was bothering me didn't help things either. We took her home that evening, and I was amazed at how well things went and how she was actually comfortable around me. Because we had known each other before I was burned, I believe it helped her see past the scars for who

I was inside. After the low points of late eighth grade and my difficulties in high school, it seemed as if things might be looking brighter.

My relationship with Amanda took off faster than I would have expected. Maybe too fast for some, but I was happy that I finally had somebody after thinking for so long that it would never happen for me. In our private chats early on, I told her about how bad I was feeling at times and suicidal thoughts. But that's all they were, just thoughts. I was never serious about suicide for many reasons. I honestly wasn't selfish enough to leave my family and friends behind, and suicide was like admitting failure and not being strong enough. Suicide would mean all the pain, time, effort, and even money was all for nothing. I wouldn't let that happen. I was strong enough to get through another day, yet like every human being, I had my low points. I was constantly thinking of Amanda, and if she couldn't come over for a day on weekends, then I tried to go to her. I think it was December 23 when I was at her place, hanging out for the evening. We were both in the kitchen, and she was rummaging through cupboards, finding stuff to eat and every so often stopped to give me a kiss. We continued this little "game," and I started to think *maybe* we're both testing the waters. So thinking it was a mistake, I just barely "pushed further" as she kissed me yet again. To my surprise, she didn't seem bothered at all, but I wondered if she even noticed. After the snack, we were sitting on the couch when the subject came up somewhat bluntly. I simply told her I had never French-kissed before and I had no idea how. She seemed dumbfounded that I had never done it before and tried to explain just how it was done. Then it happened. I won't kiss and tell, but the feelings inside just made me feel like a million bucks. I think that night was also the same night she asked me to go steady, yet another surprise. When Vicki picked me up, Amanda flat out told her I had my first kiss that night. I couldn't believe she said that and immediately assumed I might be in trouble. I actually wasn't, and on our ride home, Vicki just laughed and asked if I had a good time. I continued to spend as much time with Amanda during Christmas break as I possibly could. On the weekend, we went to Grandpa Reed's house in Pekin, she and Zachary even came along. Having a girlfriend with me made it seem like others saw me differently. I couldn't help but think having a girlfriend made me feel more like a normal person or average teenager and, needless to say, more my age. Almost like the transitional feeling when somebody gets married or has kids. Even Vicki's nieces were surprised I had a girlfriend, and Kyle tried to keep them out of his grandpa's basement so Amanda and I could have privacy on the couch. Nothing happened, and we simply cuddled up and watched TV. When Christmas arrived a few days after that party, I gave Amanda a bracelet with my name on it and the extra Simba I had from Disney after David "abused" it. She gave me a necklace with the words, "Somebody loves me," which to this day I still keep in my drawer. For so long, I had hoped that I would find somebody to fall in love with, and it finally seemed to be happening for me. For all those years prior, I had begun to assume having a girlfriend would just be another joy in life I miss out on. Life is difficult alone, and having a loved one to share life's experiences and cuddle with on cold nights are among life's best moments. For Christmas that year, I think I was so distracted by my new and growing relationship that I didn't really ask for much, and I don't remember much of it, except the stereo I received from Bob and Diane and my plasma lightning ball. I was always a lightning freak and obsessed with storm watching to the point most would call foolish or crazy. I would go outside under the porch to watch thunderstorms, but having stainless-steel hooks for hands meant it wasn't the best idea, but I still love lightning.

After Christmas, the initial fervor to constantly think of or be around Amanda had at least calmed down a little. I went with her to the school dance in Farmington, but for whatever reason, we didn't stay long and left before hardly anyone had arrived. To be honest, I was kind of relieved because dances and especially large crowds just aren't my thing. Who knows how stressed I would have been around old classmates from Farmington and Yates City. We still saw each other when we could, but I didn't seem so obsessed as early on. The Wells had gotten a second foster kid sometime around the holidays. His name was Eric, and during respite stays at Vicki's, he always hung out with Jason. Jason was the newest foster kid living with us and was only a few months older than me. Eric and Jason both had problems listening, but I honestly thought Eric wasn't so bad. I remember one day when Eric was in trouble for making out with his girlfriend in the theater and then said, "Caper doesn't get in trouble for it." Diane quickly said, "Well, Caper does it privately at home and not in a public theater." He apologized to me for that and something else he did, but not long after that, things suddenly went downhill during another respite weekend. Jason was in trouble for something gross and completely wrong. So later that night, after everyone went to bed, he and Eric quietly got up stole whatever money they could around the house, including my jar of loose change I was saving, then stole the truck and took off. What surprised Vicki is that they were dumb enough to steal a truck with big bold lettering on the side that read Bill Robinson Construction. I actually don't remember the sign and always assumed the truck was Lee's daily vehicle, but it was later found abandoned in the Quad Cities. And neither Jason nor Eric ever came back. So much was going on at this time it's hard to pinpoint exactly when important dates occurred. Vicki told me Bridgeway only allowed two kids other than me, so with Jason gone, a spot was open for my sister Cassandra. She moved in because her former foster parents were forced to move to Kansas for a job with the railroad. One date I can be sure of was the weekend of March 3. I remember the exact date easily because *Lion King* was released on video and Bob and Lee were watching us that weekend while Vicki and Diane went on a trip. Diane told me early on that I was supposed to share the video with everyone, which was fine by me and simple enough request. I planned to watch it in my room first, then everyone else could watch as much as they wanted to on the living room TV. I wanted the first time watching at home to be on my own TV, because it had closed captioning. The living room TV was an older model and thus didn't have it. Anyway, when it was over, I was eager to take the tape into my own room and begin watching it. But Bob said it had to be watched in the living room. I was annoyed and frustrated, and I wasn't being selfish or greedy in my opinion. I simply wanted to watch it with closed captioning while keeping it fresh by not watching it till then. So while mostly everyone except Kyle and Mike watched it, I waited till I could watch it in my room. When it was over, I assumed I could then finally watch it on my own TV. But for some reason which was beyond my grasp for logic, I couldn't. So I was pissed off, Bob was angry, Kyle's anger was fueling my own, and it just didn't seem fair. I let everyone have a turn, but I couldn't have my turn on my own TV. I just didn't see what the big deal was and why I was being denied watching it with closed captioning. Other than going to a movie theater, I still don't care to watch anything without closed captioning. Our anger wasn't helping the situation. Kyle fueled my frustrations, and I said, "Bob is taking this parenting crap too far." But unlike Kyle, when I was angry, I didn't talk back like he did. I let it be known I was angry or frustrated and I cussed a bit, but I didn't talk back or stand my ground, yelling pointlessly. Nope, instead, I typically went to my room and let my anger out somehow until it cooled down.

Other than the incident at school with Ryan A. and a few other not-so-bad incidents, there was one other in particular that happened around midyear. But this one, honest to God, was a simple misunderstanding on both parts. One day I was waiting between the outer and inner doors for Carl to come back over from the elementary building. As I waited, the high school custodian came up behind me and asked if I wanted or needed help getting back in. I told him I was waiting for Carl, and that was it, or so I thought. Later on that day, I was called to Principal Kernagis's office, and I had no idea why. He talked for a few minutes, and because I couldn't hear him very well, I assumed I was in trouble for cussing at another student during lunch. Ironically, the student was the custodian's son, and that's initially what I assumed I was in trouble for. But I was actually being questioned because the custodian thought I had said something inappropriate to him. I actually have no idea what it was, so when I got home that afternoon, Vicki cleared things up further and said the principal gave me the benefit of the doubt. Over the years in many situations, there would be occasions where I couldn't stand up for myself or offer input because I couldn't hear enough of what was going on to actually offer any defense or alibi. Supposedly there was a major incident that first year after, I didn't hear something said about me. I do know his name, but what happened and what he might have said I have no idea, but Kyle told Lee who, then did "something" about it. I actually didn't learn of any of it until years later, and even then, Kyle left out the actual details. Keep in mind though that Kyle sometimes started trouble just to do so. So that's why I was surprised when I heard who that student was, because as far as I knew, he never gave me any trouble at school. Being in a wheelchair *and* hard of hearing made defending myself difficult, and things would be more difficult during my sophomore year. Late that spring, I came home from school to find my crappy hospital-style bed gone and a rather large waterbed in its place. The old bed fit along the wall and left the middle of the room open. Unfortunately, the waterbed was so big it took up the majority of the room, but the comfort was worth the loss of space. More change was happening at the Wells house in Canton too. They had just gotten or were about to get another foster kid when they decided to renovate their house. Over the next few years, they would add two new bedrooms and make the kitchen and bathroom bigger. They told me it would be easier for me afterward because of the increased space. And it meant I could possibly bring my power chair when I stayed.

With a little over a month or so of school left, I unfortunately once again went back down to Galveston for more reconstructive surgery. Unlike the previous year, this one would be more painful and difficult. The year before when I went a week without solid food was torturous in its own way, but not so much physically painful as this one would be. The surgery was another axilla release of both arms. Basically, the surgery was meant to minimize the scar contractures in the armpit area which would make movement easier. I had gone through the surgery at least twice before, and it was easier said than done. I was told every time a surgery was redone that the surgeon had to go deeper into the tissue. I actually didn't find out till sometime later when another surgery was about to be redone. But with the axilla release, it's the entire process altogether that made it so painful and stressful. After the surgery, I was stuck in bed for a week or so while my arms remained wrapped and unmovable to hold them in place at shoulder level. Also, at the time, unfortunately, I was still dealing with bathroom-related issues, and it played a part in how bad I felt, and that year, Vicki had to go home while I was still stuck in bed. Feeling somewhat sick and bedridden was bad enough, but my time in Galveston that year was tough because I was more homesick than usual. I remember a few tears on my cheeks one day when the nurses were performing my daily wound care and changing my bedding. One of them said something rude and the opposite of why I had tears on my face. I was thinking of home, Amanda, high school, and how the average fifteen-year-old couldn't comprehend what I go through constantly. I thought of how my life was so different compared to everyone else back home. I lay there pretty much helpless while everyone else at home and school went about their day oblivious to what's become a normal life routine for me since I was burned five years before. Sometimes a person needs somebody to talk to or even just a friendly face in the room as a distraction from the loneliness. One day in particular, the music therapist stopped by my room and asked if I needed anything. I asked her if she would play my Bon Jovi tape for me, and when the first ballad came on, I couldn't fight the sadness.

> I'd hold you
> I'd need you
> I'd get down on my knees for you
> And make everything alright
> If you were in these arms
> I'd love you
> I'd please you
> I'd tell you that I'd never leave you
> And love you till the end of time
> If you were in these arms tonight

I never forgot that day how that music therapist, whose name I don't remember, and how she sat and listened with me as I fought and failed to fight back the tears. It was a simple moment, but for me, it was powerful because I was a human being who needed nothing else but human kindness when I felt the most alone. After the wrapping was removed and I was allowed to be up and in my wheelchair, I still had to wear airplane splints during the day for a few days. Airplane splits basically held my arms in abduction at shoulder level. They are called airplane splints because it gives the appearance of having wings like an airplane. Better than calling them birdy splints, I guess. I was told that a few folks back at school were wondering how I was and when I would be back, but the truth was I wouldn't be back in time to finish out the school year. When I no longer had to wear the splints during the day, I was then required to wear round foam inserts under my armpits to help prevent the scars contracting. I also had to have daily therapy to stretch my arms as much as possible to keep flexibility and movement, thus further limiting the contracting. The entire process was annoying, but the worst part by far was wearing the airplane splints all night. They were extremely uncomfortable and would be a major pain in the ass over the course of the next few months. Strangely, one funny thing I remember about being in Galveston that year was Vicki and I going to Walmart before we went back home. The funny part to me was actually the fact that's when I got my first pair of jeans after being burned. Initially, we both had concerns on whether I could fit and wear them comfortably. Technically, they were jean shorts, but I felt like a different person in them when I wore them to go home. It was like switching gears from pajamas to normal day clothes. To this day, I still feel naked when I'm forced to wear anything but my jeans. That's the funny aspect of it, I guess. After wearing nothing but gym shorts and summer shorts, switching to jeans made the old shorts feel out of place, as if jeans are formal wear.

When I finally got back home after a month in Galveston, school had just ended or was almost over. Just a few days before I returned, there was an outbreak of tornados in the Midwest, and one of them ravaged parts of Knox County between Hermon and Maquon. Maquon suffered minor damage here and there, but a few rural areas west of town were harder hit. Not long after I got back home, I saw firsthand the extent of the damage. I had been fortunate enough that I had never seen the results of Mother Nature at its worst. Just north of Hermon, an entire farm shed full of equipment was obliterated. Further east on the damage path, there was a combine that had been picked up and tossed down a hill, and not far from that location, there was a house that was completely destroyed. Its backside faced a steep hill, and the front of it faced the road, and just across from it was a steep ditch. The damage was as if a bomb blew up directly behind the house and the debris was blasted directly into the ditch across the road. Even though I am curious to see a tornado in person, I have recurring nightmares of finally seeing one. There was nothing left of the house except a few bricks of the foundation. I'd like to see a tornado someday, but it's not worth somebody losing their life or home. Even though I was home and summer had begun, I still had trouble adjusting to sleeping at night with those damn airplane splints. Getting comfortable and moving around to a cozy sleeping position was hard enough without the splints, let alone with them. My sleep patterns got to the point where Vicki requested a nurse to sleep over and help as needed during the night. So Mary, a nurse from Spoon River Home Health, began sleeping nights. That went well. (Insert sarcasm.) Those splints drove me nuts. It was next to impossible for me to get comfortable enough to sleep, which only frustrated me and reached a point where it all just started to piss me off. I only wanted to sleep, but those splints were an obstacle, and I was to be stuck with them for at least six months. I don't remember how, but Mary didn't last that long as everyone's frustration increased as time dragged on. Therapists were seeing me occasionally to keep my progress steady, but I'm being completely honest when I say that with each new therapist over the years, something had been lost in the translation so to speak. With each passing therapist, the therapy just seemed to lack the proper technique. I know how effective my home therapy was compared to Lindbergh, Methodist, and Shriners, but I was forced to stick with it even though I mostly felt it lagged behind in effectiveness and proper technique.

Chapter 26

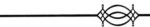

Summer of '95 was busier than usual, and with a lot going on, I can't be sure who or what came first. Early in the summer one day, while everyone else was on the trampoline, I was speeding down the sidewalk in front of the house. When I reached the corner of the sidewalk, as my left front tire hit the corner, my wheelchair came to a dead stop, and I was suddenly airborne. I fell legs first onto the sidewalk then slammed my head. Kyle saw what happened as I lay there grimacing and shaking from the intense pain and adrenaline. Vicki rushed out, and most people are usually worried about my head, but even though I'd never fallen or flipped a chair before, my main concern was actually my legs. My legs had hit first, and they have little to no muscle mass to soften the blow, so that impact goes straight to solid bone, which meant it hurt like hell. To make matters worse, the initial impact was at the worst possible part of my legs, the very end where the bone takes the brunt of the force. Vicki picked me up and put me back in my chair, and even though I was still shaken up and obviously bruised, I appeared to be okay. But not long afterward, I noticed a sharp piercing pain in my right leg whenever I moved a certain way. Vicki decided I needed to be checked out, and we went to St. Mary's ER in Galesburg. We waited forever, but the hardest part was actually the X-ray. I went in without Vicki, and because the

X-ray table was too hard, my body and muscles stiffened when I was laid on it, which triggered the pain in my leg. The doctors told Vicki and me I had broken my leg and would probably need a cast. I don't remember the details, but Vicki and I didn't quite agree and sought a second opinion from ER doctors at good old Methodist in Peoria. All I remember from that visit was simply being told that I fractured my femur but a cast wasn't needed, so that was that. But later that summer, I ended up visiting Methodist ER again, but that time, it wasn't my fault. For some reason, my power wheelchair was out of commission again, and Vicki began running as she pushed my wheelchair down the sidewalk. I had just told her to slow down when the chair hit a bump, and down we went with Vicki cartwheeling over me. She felt bad because she was worried of reinjuring my femur, but luckily, I was fine. I had learned my lesson the first time, and I haven't fallen or hurt myself since, and Vicki learned not to run with my wheelchair.

So much was going on I can't remember what came first. But Vicki's brother Wally ended up moving in during the summer. Vicki bought him a small used trailer for only $100, which he slept in. He was always trying to convince me to loan him my TV for his camper, but then I wouldn't have anything to do during the day. Eventually, one night I decided to sleep in the camper. I don't know why I was drawn to it, but I enjoyed sleeping in it. It really didn't make much sense because the sleeping space was tiny, the bed was rather hard, no color TV, Wally snored, and every morning, I was carried back inside for my shower. Despite the inconvenience of sleeping in the camper, I still enjoyed it, and I can't explain why. I won't go into details, but at about the same time Wally moved in, I had somewhat of a success moment when I fully regained control of my "personal" bodily functions, which meant one less thing to worry about. Joey spent the night quite a bit, which helped alleviate my summer boredom, but there wasn't really a lot of inactivity when compared to other summers. In the middle of the summer, Vicki made a spur-of-the-moment decision to take us to Six Flags again. Only this time she did it alone with at least seven or eight kids all in one day and without staying at a hotel if I remember correctly. I remember Vicki was worried about Alisha aggravating her broken wrist or getting the cast wet. She walked around the park with it wrapped in plastic, but that was pointless because it still ended up getting wet. My favorite memory from that visit happened during one of the stage performances. The show was a mix of country singers and Chinese acrobatic performers. At one point, one of the costumed Chinese dragons approached Michael, and his reaction was hilarious. He acted like a five-year-old and yelled an incoherent squeal of "Ehhhhh." He was always like that. Quick to mouth off and just as quick to run away like a scared cat surrounded by a pack of dogs. But there was one particular weekend when everyone else but me had gotten in trouble for smoking. Dustin was with us that weekend, and I was disappointed to hear that even he had supposedly been part of it. The accused had all been across the street, and each denied and blamed the others involved. Because I had no part of it, I had the privilege of being taken to the movies by our neighbors. I think that was also the weekend I went to my first *Star Trek* convention. My grandma was with me, but strangely, that was the one occasion that stands out in my memory of Vicki taking me to such an event. Sure, we went shopping, parks, museums, etc. but not a personal interest such as *Star Trek*. Even though it was incredibly small compared to conventions elsewhere, that was the first time I met an actor. *Star Trek: Voyager* had started its first season a few months before after its predecessor was cancelled. And one of the most important characters was the hologram doctor played by Robert Picardo. I always liked his character because he always strived to evolve and better himself as a person even though his character was actually a hologram. As I approached him after being in line for his autograph, I quietly thanked him and was on my way. At the time, I think I was just too shy to say much more than that, but in the future, some actors I met would be quieter than others or simply too focused or too tired to really say much. But a few actually took extra time to converse, and either way, I always thanked them for signing and for coming.

Summer of 1995 I remember mostly as summer of the ducks. By then, Bob and Diane had another boy staying with them named Ken. He was kind of quiet and tall, but a little awkward. Every kid Vicki or the Wells had always had problems, but Ken actually wasn't too bad compared to all the crap I'd seen over the years. Anyway, the Wells went on a trip to Mississippi, and they took along Michael while Ken stayed with us. I think I remember asking them to bring back some pet ducks, but I truly honestly didn't think they actually would. When they arrived back home to pick up Ken, they said they had something outside, and there I saw two little ducklings swimming in a steel tub. I couldn't believe they actually brought ducks back for me. They said they had to stop constantly on the way home to feed and water them. I was excited because I had wanted ducks for years ever since my grandma almost got us some for Easter back in 1988. I loved those ducks, and they grew fast. Initially, we kept them inside in a wire cage down in the basement while they were still small, and then when they were big enough, we put them in a round wire pen outside. If I was outside, I was usually watching them or helping others find grasshoppers to feed them. They loved the grasshoppers as well as the feeder fish and minnows I got for them occasionally. Every time we poured the fish in their kiddie pool, they went nuts until every fish was devoured. Sometimes we would take them out to the grass field so they could stretch their wings and enjoy the open space, and that's when we learned they would fly home if they took off. The smaller one, which I named Darkwing, flew and landed perfectly in the pool. The brownish and bigger duck, which I named Daisy, wasn't so good at landing and always seemed to crash head-first, plowing into the ground. They never left the yard, and they were never in any danger, so eventually, as they got older, I let them out of their pen for a few hours a day to enjoy the grass. I don't know whose idea it was, but Darrin, Kyle, and I participated in a lip sync contest that summer in London Mills. The song was "Fat Little Baby" by Amy Grant and was chosen by Darrin. Darrin was a great singer and actor, so he played the role of singer while Kyle was the husband and I played the role of his hangout buddy. We practiced for days with Darren perfecting his routine while Kyle and I played our simple parts by acting annoyed with his nagging wife. We did three lip sync contests that summer. The first one obviously was in London Mills, and we won simply because of the lack of competition. It was easy money even if it was only $17 after we divided it between us. When we did our second contest in Elmwood, we weren't so fortunate. We had more kids competing against us, and the crowd was much larger. Later, we learned that somebody from DCFS found out that I participated in the contest and tried to keep me from doing so in the future. A few months before that, I was talking to Clare Howard from the *Peoria Journal Star* because she was interested in doing a story about me, but she was denied after DCFS found out about it. Supposedly they thought Vicki was trying to parade me in front of people or show me off somehow. I was angry because I felt they had no right to tell me what I couldn't do. They didn't own me, and I still talked to the press pretty much every year at camp while I was still under eighteen and in foster care.

Summer of 1995 was also the only year Kyle and I both had to attend summer school. He had missed a few weeks of school due to his own personal issues, and I obviously missed the final month of school. The only other year I attended summer school was back in 1989 after moving back and forth between Colorado and Illinois. In my opinion, the summer school session at Valley was pointless. It was barely a half-day session and seemed more like punishment than anything else. It wasn't torturous like actual detention but very boring, and I read books more than anything else. I didn't mind reading, but I could do that at home if I wanted to, but summer was the one time of year when you are supposed to be free of the chains of enslavement known as school. Late that summer before camp was also the big incident I had with

Vicki's mom, Elaine. Vicki, Lee, Diane, and Bob all went to Wisconsin one weekend while Elaine and Wally stayed home with us. The house was full of kids, including Michael and Ken. Everything was fine until lunch one day. Everybody was eating sandwiches or whatever, and I simply said I wasn't that hungry, and I think I didn't want something put on my plate. I don't remember what it was, but she immediately overreacted and seemed to forget I was old enough to make my own choices. I was almost sixteen years old, and because of my appearance, some people tend to forget or ignore that fact. It all went downhill quickly, and for me, my anger point shot up when she said, "Now I see what your mom is talking about if you guys always act like this." I was pissed because she dared compare my behavior at that moment to anyone else. I may have cussed sometimes, but I guarantee you, so did every other teenager, and even then, not as much as Kyle did. I never hit, stole things, ran away, talked back, got arrested, smoked, or did drugs, like any number of kids in that house, and she dared compare me to Kyle? Kyle was also in trouble for something, though I don't remember what. Over the years, Kyle did a lot of stuff, some I don't remember and some I do, but for the most part, I'm not going to list every single offense of his. We are all human, we all make mistakes, and it's in the past. But nonetheless, once she made that remark, she lost my respect. I'm sure that loss of respect was mutual, but I honestly didn't care. What I did hardly warranted the reaction and punishment that followed. I don't know if Vicki or anyone else complained about me sometimes, but I actually hated it whenever I was called a troublemaker or anything similar. I have always assumed that all those troublemaker rumors that surround me are the reason some people out there and at school don't take the time to get to know me and just assume the worst about me. But as I mentioned above, I never did anything overtly bad, not even in school. I had one detention my entire four years in high school, and I bet Kyle couldn't even count how many he had, let alone how many physical fights he got into. I never got into fights, I didn't smoke, I wasn't mean, etc. Some people only see my faults and my biggest would be my cussing, but that hardly made me a bad person. So her comparing me to any of the other kids in the house highly offended me and showed me how ignorant she was of the kind of person I really am inside.

Near the end of August, just before school, camp was again upon us. That year, I remember during the ride up to camp we listened to my *Lion King* soundtrack full blast in the van. It felt weird with a van full of teenagers listening to "Hakuna Matata," but I admit it was a good weird. Joey and I still laugh at the bathroom incident when we stopped at McDonald's in DeKalb that year. The other boys were laughing in the bathroom as Joey helped me out. He was slightly annoyed at the laughs, so suddenly, without warning, he threw the urinal I had just used over the bathroom stall to get them to shut up. He laughed, and they scattered, so I guess you could say it worked, and though I felt sorry for any other customers walking in there before it was cleaned up, at least it didn't hit anyone. That year, my cabin was Woodpecker and more or less had all the same guys I was with the year before. On visitors' day, I remember Joey's foster care caseworker butting in when I was talking to somebody from the press. I couldn't help but think the only reason she was there was to solely prevent Joey and me from being interviewed for any articles, but she couldn't be there all week, and there was plenty of chances that year and in the future to do so. What stands out most about camp being special that year was meeting Mara Koonsvitsky Heichman. I asked her to write a little something because I feel it's important to include the perspective of my story as seen by other people.

In her words: "I was working as an occupational therapist in the health center at burn camp. I had been working as an OT at the burn unit at Loyola University Medical Center for a little over a year at that point. I had seen numerous significant burn injuries and met many resilient people, but meeting Caper was an absolute experience and one I will never forget. He was scarred from head to toe and missing parts of all of his limbs. He required lotion, massage, stretching, and wound care while he was at camp. Not to mention an escape from the extreme heat. Because of all of this, he spent a lot of time in the health center, and we got to know each other very quickly and very intimately. We spent a lot of time on the back floor of the health center, caring for his wounds and scars, but the most important thing we did back there was talk and connect—for hours. We talked about everything from *Star Wars*, Bon Jovi, and cars, of course, to our hopes and dreams. Caper was always filled with humor and optimism and yet had a realistic spin on everything.

"When I first met Caper, he had difficulty feeding himself, turning himself, and using the washroom. Because I only got to see him once a year back then, I would see him improve his skills by leaps and bounds each year. His progress and determination was truly inspirational. At one point, he even came back to camp with prosthetic legs and walker and took several steps. My friendship with Caper is one I can't explain like other friendships. We are bonded like I'm bonded with no other friend. He holds a place in my heart, and I'm so grateful for his friendship."

Because of my needs, we spent a lot of time together and forged a strong friendship. Through all the years at camp, there have been plenty of memories made, but there are always special moments that stand out above the rest. Almost every year we go back, Mara mentions how much fun she had playing capture the flag with me. Before the game started, we had our faces painted to identify which team we were on, and Mara still keeps a photo, a memory of that moment. She would freak out every time the opposing team made a run for our flag. While she was screaming in terror, I was just laughing at the sight of her doing so. That week at camp was just the beginning of our friendship, and it grew as the years passed. We all have people who fill holes or niches in our lives, and Mara was like that for me. I borrowed a quote from Jon Bon Jovi when he said, "She's my best friend, my mother, my girlfriend, and my sister, all in one," and I'm truly thankful to have such a kind person as a friend. Camp was always replenishment for my heart and soul. Every time camp was over, I felt renewed and ready to overcome the obstacles in my way. Any worries and stresses of typical daily burn survivor life are less of a concern when I had everlasting friendships and support from all of my camp family. But unfortunately, my sophomore school year ahead would be my most difficult in more ways than one.

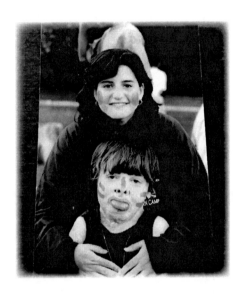

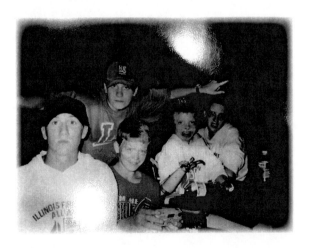

Chapter 27

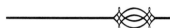

I did spend a little time now and then with Amanda during the summer. But sometime between her birthday in August and mine, she called me one day, and to put it bluntly, we were quietly breaking up. Neither of us had done anything wrong, and we were still getting along just fine. She told me she had thought about it for a while, and even her high school counselor told her she needed to think of her future and her son Zachary. In her words, she said, "She couldn't take care of Zachary and me at the same time." Then she talked about how she was worried about how I might react and was afraid I might slip into a depression or even suicide. When we first got together, I told her about my low points before we met and how rough things had been off and on. She said we would stay friends as I told her truthfully and honestly I didn't blame her for needing to end it. I agreed with her though that Zachary needed to come first, and I would not come between them. What kind of selfish person would I be if I had? Somebody had to be there for him, and his own mom was that person. She was upset, and I tried to calm her down and assure her I was okay, and initially, I mostly was. But as time passed over the weeks and months, those thoughts and feelings changed. Still, I never blamed her for anything; it just wasn't meant to be, but that didn't make it any easier. I tried to rationalize why it ended. Life circumstances, challenges, difficulties, responsibilities, her son, and future children. Vicki had told me Amanda asked all kinds of personal questions, including whether or not I could still father any kids. I sometimes wondered if she had only asked me herself if it might have influenced her decision. Then along with the eventual depression also came anger. Anger that she assumed I would need to be cared for and unable to contribute or provide anything. But the anger was just a natural defense against the depression and part of the long healing process. Early on, I was okay when we first split, but as time went on, my depression set in, and even though I tried to hide it and keep it to myself, Vicki eventually noticed a change in my personality and asked just what my problem was. Music and alone time were my methods of self-therapy. Joey spending the night, shopping, or other fun boosted my spirits, but it was always temporary. I spent a lot of time listening to Bon Jovi ballads as I just wondered where it all went. Not just my relationship with Amanda, but my life in those five years since I had been burned so much had changed. So many of his songs spoke directly to me and seemed to mirror almost exactly what I was going through. Even though so many of his songs echoed my emotions, here are three examples of what I listened to.

I Want You

I never wanted the stars
Never shot for the moon
I like them right where they are
All I wanted was you
So baby just turn away
Because I can't face the truth
All I'm trying to say
Is all I wanted was you
I tried so hard to remember

When where how why love went away
I tried to drown myself in pity
But her memory kept calling my name, yes it did

Lie to Me

If you don't love me—lie to me
'Cause baby you're the one thing I believe
Let it all fall down around us, if that's what's
meant to
Right now if you don't love me baby—lie to me

I'll Be There for You

You say you've cried a thousand rivers
And now you're swimming for the shore
You left me drowning in my tears
And you won't save me anymore
Now I'm praying to God you'll give me one
more chance, girl

I'll be there for you
These five words I swear to you
When you breathe I want to be the air for you
I'll be there for you
I'd live and I'd die for you
Steal the sun from the sky for you
Words can't say what a love can do
I'll be there For you.

Aside from my personal struggles though there was one thing that made eating easier and faster. Sometime over the summer I had adapted to eating without using the clunky eating. Not only did it help at school but it made all meals easier, faster, less messy, and I even eventually learned to eat sandwiches myself without it falling to pieces. As if dealing with breaking up wasn't bad enough, I also had problems at school. I was now a sophomore, and I had looked forward to Darrin being a freshman that year. Darrin, Bill Fisher, Ken Walters, and occasionally another student sat at our little round table almost every day for lunch. Kyle, unfortunately, never joined me for lunch because by then he ended up going to a different school in Canton. As far as I remember, the only class I shared with Darrin was math with Mrs. Agnoletti. That year, my favorite class was easily driver's ed. It was easy for me and seemed almost effortless. And even though I did get an A in the class, I was unable to participate in the behind-the-wheel training portion of the class simply because the school lacked the necessary adaptive equipment I required to be able to drive. As usual, math was most difficult with science replacing biology as my other difficult class. But my problems with science class were mostly due to the distractions. Ironically, with Darrin came the new freshman class, and it was a particular group of them that seemed intent on making high school harder than the previous year. Science class was the class some of them managed to bother me the most. Even Darrin being friends with almost all of them meant nothing. My own freshman class the year before never aggravated me so much as the new one, and any problems from my own class that year were actually minimal or sometimes lumped in with what the freshman might have been doing to me any particular day. Darrin tried to get them to stop and even went so far as to tell Principal Walters what was going on. His answer was he couldn't do anything about it unless one of the school faculty members saw it happen, and it was Darrin's word against his own group of friends. Such lazy, uncaring attitude, why would Darrin "narc" on his own friends if they had done nothing? It was an incident during science class that I finally reached a boiling point. That particular day, we were in the chemistry lab going over safety, protocol, and other lab stuff before we began working with the lab equipment. As Mr. Klusman lectured on and on, the usual group took advantage whenever Klusman wasn't paying attention. A few of them gave me glaring evil looks as rubber stoppers were thrown at me every time Klusman had his back turned. Rubber stoppers are the small black rubber corks used to top the glass beakers. Anyway, I was sitting there pissed off, unable to do anything, not saying anything, but wishing I wasn't stuck in that wheelchair while forced to put up with such bull crap. I had a right to an education without dealing with daily harassment from thugs who I otherwise would have confronted if not constrained by my disabilities. When the bell rang, I was eager to get away, leave for the next class, and leave them gladly behind. The group of offenders went out one by one, but I was surprised when one of them, Jeremy Miller, held the door open for me. My first thought was, did I judge him wrong? Or perhaps he was sorry for what happened. When I was about ten feet down the hallway, I was suddenly bombarded by a handful of rubber stoppers slamming the back of my head. A few students looked my way after it happened, but nobody said or did anything. At that point, I was fuming, and I had enough. I didn't care about my next class as I went back to Mrs. Fulton's room, angrily threw my books on the desk, and went straight to the secretary's office and asked her to call Vicki. During my four years at Valley, I was never so pissed off as I was at that moment. When Vicki arrived, I explained what had happened, and we both went in to talk to Principal Walters. He seemed to be less than concerned, and this is what he said to Vicki and me, "Well, Mrs. Davis, boys will be boys, and after all, look at the way your son looks. You might as well get used to it." Then she proceeded down the hall, pissed off, went into the super's office, and he recited the exact same words. It's so ironic that I had more support from the principal's son Ken than his own dad. During my freshman year, former principal Mr. Kernagis seemed like he actually wanted me there.

But when he left, everything just seemed to go downhill, and very little effort was made by the school administration to curtail the bullying and teasing. The first year, Vicki would call and talk to parents, and as far as I know, she didn't have a problem. But when she made calls to a few of the new freshman students giving me problems, Paul Stuckel's mother in particular had the gall to daresay I was bullying her son. When Vicki told me what his mom said, I was just dumbfounded. How could I be a bully to Paul when I never actually spoke a single word to him? How anyone could look at the situation and assume I was the aggressor is just unbelievable. Paul and everyone with him had strength in numbers and the physical and not to mention egotistical assertion to back them up. I was grateful I had Darrin's support and friendship during lunch hours, but there was only so much he could do.

After the incident in science class, Mr. Klusman talked to me about what happened that day in class and asked me to point out who participated. I knew most of the names, but unfortunately, there was one senior in the class whom I did misidentify. He was actually one of the few who wasn't afraid to say hello and didn't act like I was invisible. But after that incident, he acted differently around me, and I assumed it was because of me. I've long since forgotten his name, and I wish I could have apologized for the simple mistake. There was one other incident that year from that same group of students, but this time, the aggressor didn't get away with it. Darrin and I were having lunch when Nathan Allen started throwing his fries at me, but nothing could be done unless school staff saw it happen. That's when Nathan messed up and my aide Carl witnessed it. So now with the word of a school employee and Darrin as backup, we went to the office, and punishment was finally handed out in the form of a suspension. It was a small victory for me that day, knowing somebody would finally be punished for all that crap and perhaps might make them think twice in the future. Eventually, things were at least a little easier to deal with by the second semester. That made things a little less stressful and easier to focus on my classes.

For my birthday, Vicki and Diane had decided to combine parties for Michael and me because our birthdays were both in October. We both invited quite a few people, and mine was extra special because it was my sixteenth birthday. My brothers, grandparents, friends, and family were all there, and it was the biggest party I ever had. But I always found it hard to spend time with everyone when there were so many people present. We had the usual party stuff food, cake, ice cream, and of course, birthday presents. For the entertainment, Vicki had hired a magician who brought along her granddaughter. I couldn't help but think she looked very familiar, and my suspicions ended up being correct. Her name was Brandi, and she was a former classmate who left Lindbergh after my first year. It was a great party, and I received money for shopping, but most of all, it was a nice distraction from my daily life at the time. Apart from school, the drama at home eventually began to heat up again. Quiet periods at home were few, and there always seemed to be somebody acting up and causing problems. I don't remember exactly when, but Alisha went down the same path as her brother did, but instead of running away, she reacted violently one day until Vicki had to step in. Afterward, she was removed from the home, and caseworkers asked us our views of what happened. I answered honestly, and the shortened version of that answer was that Alisha basically had a violent tantrum kicking, screaming, cussing, and Vicki had to restrain her. Meanwhile, Ken had run away from the Wells, and Bobbi Joe eventually moved in. And then as if Alisha hadn't been enough, my sister eventually started acting up also. There would be just a few short times when she seemed okay, but once she had set her mind on not changing, her troubles were never-ending. During the scenic drive weekend, I enjoyed showing off my ducks to people as they browsed what we were selling that year. I let them roam free in the front yard, and people would watch and smile when they saw them. But a few weeks later, one of them vanished overnight on the same day Bob was taken to the hospital for heart troubles. Diane showed up, and I admit I was worried about my duck. Diane thought I had been more concerned with the duck than Bob, but I honestly believed he was fine. And I think part of me didn't want to believe Bob's health could be something serious. As the season grew colder, the lone duck noticeably changed. He seemed to miss his companion and was friendlier when we were near him, but unfortunately, he too ended up vanishing one night.

Back at school, around November or so, I went on a field trip to Chicago to the art institute and the field museum. Ever since I was up there that day, I have wanted to go back and spend time up there without being rushed or chaperoned by school staff. Plus, I appreciate art and history even more now than I did then. I liked history, but as I got older, I learned to appreciate art history and architectural history as well. Before the trip, I had considered calling Scott, Mike, or even Mara to see if they might meet up to say hello. Part of me wanted to show off to everyone else that I indeed have a social life that included adult friends from the Chicago area, but I decided against it. I figured somebody might question my judgment of meeting up with a friend on what was supposed to be an educational field trip. Still, I couldn't help but think if they only knew I had been in town that day. Apart from dealing with the freshman class, there was one more unpleasant incident that first semester. But this one was different because it was simply a stroke of extremely bad luck on my part. I was in Mrs. Fulton's room one day, and I noticed something about how she looked at me. The bell rang, I left her room, and she just smiled at me as I went to math class. On my way there, literally the entire school laughed, pointed, and stared as I proceeded to math class, but I had no idea why. It wasn't until I parked in front of Darrin in math class when he whispered to me that my sweat shorts and part of my underwear had slipped down almost to my knees. I didn't know they had slipped off because I still used a lapboard across the armrests of my chair. The lapboard made it impossible to see anything under it, and I couldn't feel any difference when they slipped off. I was mortified and by then well aware that the entire class and most of the school knew of my humiliation. Even Mrs. Agnoletti was aware but seemed just as frozen as I was to do anything about it. After deciding I had enough, I bravely and quietly asked to be excused and then left class to find Carl, who then helped me correct the problem. I did not and could not face my class after that and simply waited for lunch. I don't know what I would have done if Darrin had not been there to tell me. So thank God he was there for me, but it could have been prevented if Mrs. Fulton had said something in the first place instead of just smiling at me when I left her room. A little courtesy would have been much appreciated in that situation, but instead, I was fed to the wolves. I had enough problems without handing them extra ammunition.

I spent Thanksgiving with Bob and Diane that year, partly to avoid going with Vicki to her mom's. I still preferred it with the Wells anyway, because I could always expect the classic food, and it wasn't so crowded. Fast forward a month to Christmas, and we went to all the usual parties and got our tree at Grady's tree farm again. That was either the first or second year our foster care party was at a buffet in Galesburg. Even though it was a bit crowded for me, I still looked forward to it because it gave us more time than usual at the buffet. We could eat, relax a bit, and go back for more compared to a normal visit where we just go in and out like any other place. But the party that year was annoying for me, at least because Vicki made up her own Christmas song for our caseworker Samantha and expected us to sing it. I love Christmas, but I didn't enjoy being expected to per-form like a trained seal. Voluntary and forced are two different things. That's the difference between the previous lip sync contests and the Christmas song. Sometimes people forget I wasn't a little kid any-more, but because of my size and appearance, I was still treated that way occasionally. Cassandra's problems seemed to worsen because either during or after Christmas was her first time she was caught shoplifting. Everything that went on in that home affected me in one way or another. Cassandra is my sister, and I just wish she could have stayed out of trouble. I only wanted what was best for her. One of my theories for her behavior was simply not being able to adjust to rules. At home, Mom couldn't control them, and they got away with a lot. But now, some of my siblings struggled to adapt to that change, and Cassandra was the one who seemed to struggle most. I think she believed if she was bad enough that she would go home, but it didn't work that way. I liken Christmas that year to that of a kid who had seen *Star Wars* and dreamed of a new Millennium Falcon under the tree. Okay, maybe it wasn't quite magical as that, but I had hoped to see it waiting for me. Vicki had agreed to get it for my birthday, but it arrived weeks later, and after Peggy helped me open the shipping package, Vicki was pissed off. By the way, Peggy was a friend of Wally's who would eventually be the family nanny to help Vicki out. Naturally, I assumed the gift was still for my birthday, but to my disappointment, she said she was sending it back. I was relieved when I still got it for Christmas but would rather have avoided the prior misunderstanding and frustration in the first place. Dustin eventually visited during the holidays too, and by then, his sister Ashley had just started visiting again after growing old enough and realizing she didn't need to be scared of me. Of all the kids who were ever scared of me then got past it, Ashley seemed to change most. It was as if even when we had just met, she was never scared of me in the first place.

With early spring came more big changes. At home, we had a girl from Farmington named Shannon, who was staying with us during afternoon and evening hours until she could go home. The reason for her time with us was because she was about to have a baby and would be staying with us off and on for a few months. Also, about that time, Vicki opened a small crafts and antique business called the Old Oak Tree just a short ways west of Farmington. Prior to that, Vicki and Lee used that location as a rental home for extra income but decided to turn it into a business and allow Wally to stay there. Vicki doesn't remember, but sometime during the spring, Alisha also moved back in. It seemed okay for a short while, but it wouldn't last. One night when Bobbi Joe and Michael were staying over for respite weekend, Alisha and Cassandra had been in trouble for something and told Bobbi Jo they were running away that night. But it backfired when she didn't join them, and we found out the next morning what had happened. They were both found, and this time Alisha was gone for good, but my sister's problems had only begun. Cassandra was becoming increasingly convinced that she was a victim in a cruel home, and it only got worse as time went on. The more lies she told about how things were, the more I was pissed off because she was trying to paint herself as a victim. She just never took any responsibility for her own actions and blamed everything and anything. My depression over my breakup had just started to ease up by that time. I had started seeing a social worker whose name was Rusty Orwig, and he was actually a severe-burn survivor like me. I was initially nervous about meeting him, but we actually got along pretty well. We talked about all sorts of things, like my hobbies, high school, moving on past hard times, and my hopes for the future. Even though I had no real interest in it, we also talked about hunting with his crossbow. But he never did show it to me like he said he would. School, on the other hand, was a little easier during the second semester, but the very start of it was marred by a student death just as Christmas break ended. Teenagers all too often think they are invincible. They think it won't happen to them, but it can, and it will. One generation learns its lesson the painfully hard way, and the very next repeats the mistake because the past lesson had already faded. The mistake was one that many are familiar with, and even with all the warnings and dangers, they do it anyway. The mistake was underage drinking and driving, and the consequence was a needless death. After the harassment and distractions of the first semester, I went from a near failing grade in science to at least a B grade, if I remember correctly. The teasing didn't stop altogether, but it eased up enough that I could focus on the class. On the last day of the school year, I assumed I would be allowed to stay home and let my report card arrive by mail. A big part of wanting to stay home was simply because I missed the last day of school the year before and I actually didn't know what to expect. I did hear rumors of water fights, but since I didn't ride the bus, I had no worries about that. But mostly, I thought it was pointless to get up early for only an hour or so of time at school just to pick up a report card. It went smoothly until I was told I had to pay a fine for drawing on my science book. It wasn't on the cover; it was actually on the exposed edge of the combined pages. I had seen other books the same way, and it didn't impede its function, but I was still fined anyway. So I had to call Vicki because my fine had to be paid before I was given my report card. I don't remember if Vicki came immediately or not, but my entire morning at school was pretty much pointless. I could've gotten more done by getting an early start on my '96 summer vacation. Of all the summers during my time in high school, that one stands out fondly as my favorite. Initially, Rusty was the person who helped me begin to move on past my depression. But in early June, I became friends with a dude who I consider a brother, and he very much helped me move past the difficulties I experienced all year.

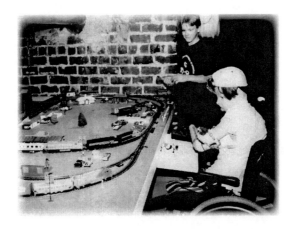

Chapter 28

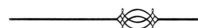

About a month before camp, yet another foster child moved in. His full name was Francisco Ceja, but everyone called him Paco. Most foster kids always came and went without blinking an eye. Many of them were in emergency situations where they needed temporary residence until something more permanent was found. I couldn't help but judge Paco as soon as I saw him. I assumed he was just another troubled punk drifting through foster care, and I kept my distance. Paco was the same age I was, and I didn't have a lot of luck making friends with my own age group, and I also assumed he would be gone within days and that would be the end of it. I don't remember exactly how, but after a week or two with us, we just started talking one day, and things just seemed to click between us. We shared a lot of common interests like *Star Wars*, *Transformers*, music, family, '80s toys from our childhood like Thundercats and G.I. Joe. The list was large and sparked a lot of conversations between us, which helped initially build our friendship. Heck, I even learned we lived only a few blocks apart in Galva back in the early '80s. Anyhow, I was *half* right when I assumed he would be gone before long. Every few days, he was told by his caseworker he would be moving out soon, but for whatever reason, circumstances kept changing to keep him with us just a little longer. Eventually, he did leave, and I thought that was it.

But at about the same time when Paco had left, Vicki finally gave in and let me get a Sony PlayStation with some money I had in my savings account. The newest technology was always a thrill, and the first PlayStation seemed to be light years ahead of the Sega and Nintendo systems. Ever since its release, I used every tactic I could to beg her to let me get one. Bribery, slavery, worship, and even saying it would enhance my coordination skills, which was actually true. Now that I think about it, she probably gave in because summer was arriving and I'd be spending more time indoors to avoid the hotter days. After I got the PlayStation, Paco ended up returning for a while, and his cycle of not knowing when he would truly leave for good continued on. The entire time, they told him he'd be leaving soon, and it never happened, but by the sound of it, I didn't think but was still hoping he might stick around awhile.

Burn camp 1996, there was new changes left and right. The biggest change was that they changed the date camp was held, from August to late June. IFSA staff and administration agreed that August was just too hot for the campers and especially me. Back then, the hot days were many, and the cabins did not have air conditioning. During the day, the fastest and most effective way to cool down was facilitated cooling with cool water from a cup or even straight out of a garden hose. It would still be a few years until the individual cabins got their own AC units. Also, that summer was when I finally started staying the night with Joey at the Spences'. It was a little easier on the day we left for camp because obviously it's twenty-five miles closer to the pickup spot at the Galesburg Fire Department than where I lived in Rapatee. We woke up, went for a quick breakfast at the doughnut shop, and then to the fire department, where we got in the vans, took off, and left the everyday world behind for a week. But this trip was different because the volunteers from Galesburg were no longer driving us all the way to Chicago. Instead, we picked up Josh in Pekin, and from there, we went to Bloomington and boarded a coach. I must also point out that for much of the trip we were listening to an Adam Sandler album titled *They're All Gonna Laugh at You*. And on the bus, it was no exception. That first year on the bus was the only year they actually had all the kids get off the bus for breakfast at McDonald's. It was crazy insane, but Joey and I seemed the calmest in the bunch. We obviously already ate, so we weren't really hungry. There was one annoying boy in particular about eight years old who was already hyper-excited, and he asked and actually received a cup of coffee. Joey and I were staring at each other, and we were like "Noooo way." When we got a chance, Joey spiked and ruined the kid's coffee with some salt, and thus, crisis averted. The ride up there on the coach was fun. Sometimes the TVs on board worked, but we always had other kids to talk to or room to stretch out and lay down if we got tired. The only downside was some of the buses had poor air conditioning, and it could be real torture on those hot days. It was all worth it when we got closer and finally pulled into the long private road to camp. Not only do we finally get off the bus, but we are excited to see everyone after another long year. Every year, it's the same; it starts out somewhat quiet, but the magic kicks in, and we all grow and bond together like family that's held strong for years.

The summer of '96 was my final year as a camper. I had four great years as a camper, and at sixteen years old, I had already reached the age limit, and it had me wondering what I would do when it was over. I loved coming to camp every summer, and I would miss the friendship and fun all too much if it was to end. But I heard rumors through the grape vine of a new program being started to allow former campers to become counselors. I even heard it was initially suggested just so I could continue returning, so I at least had positive hopes for returning somehow. Camp seemed much better in terms of temperature in June than in August. The heat was usually more tolerable in June, and we no longer had school waiting to start when we returned home. But there also seemed to be more thunderstorms in June. I loved watching the storms, but at camp, safety always came first, and more often than not, I couldn't get to a good storm-watching spot because it wasn't safe. That wasn't by my choice, of course. Camp operations staff had procedures in place because any injuries due to weather, especially negligent ones, could be a liability and an insurance issue. That year, Vicki came up for visitors' day, and she brought along a welcome surprise for me. She had brought up my power wheelchair for me to use that day. It was awesome to finally be mobile at camp without relying on others to push me around. Nobody at camp had seen nor knew I even had a power chair, and seeing me mobile was as new to them as it was for me to have that extra boost of independence in a place I loved to be. At the end of visitors' day, I was begging Vicki to let me keep my chair for the rest of the week. The two main problems with that were getting it back home and the simple fact that Vicki didn't bring along the charger. At home, even during the school week, it could last almost all week between charges. But camp was a large area with rolling hills, and we were constantly going from one place to another all day long for various activities, so obviously, the power drain was faster. Vicki let me keep the chair for the remainder of the week, but it indeed started to die with a day or two still left. But I enjoyed every precious minute of that freedom of mobility. Relying on others for so much really decreases the joy I get from doing simple things, and having it available just boosted my excitement and made camp that much better. The final full day of camp was always emotional. By that time, everyone was physically and mentally exhausted yet not quite ready to go home. Back then, we had the individual camper awards, cabin awards, staff awards for five years at camp, etc., and finally the graduation of the sixteen-year-olds whose time as campers was ending. As my name was called, I was proud and happy to be graduating with the guys I met and became friends with over the four years I had been attending camp. We all received IFSA watches as a graduation gift, and even though they were very nice, mine unfortunately didn't last because it had a loose hand inside. On the day of departure, everyone's emotions are boiling over, and we are sad to go. The big difference that year was the length of time we sat on the coach waiting to leave. The previous years, it was four or five of us in the van, and off we went. But now it was a coach full of kids waving and saying good-bye to each and every counselor as if to prolong avoiding the inevitable moment we had to leave. That only made some of the more emotionally stressed counselors even more so as it dragged on. But eventually, we finally left while I had my head in the window, waving *so long* as I saw a few tears from random counselors. The tears were reciprocal, felt by camper and counselor and triggered by each other as if by a mutual chain reaction. When the bus had finally hit the road for some of us, myself included, was when our sadness hit like a slap in the face. As we realized it was over, we missed particular friends and tried hard to not let the other campers see us cry too much.

When I returned from camp, my friendship with Paco grew stronger as we hung out more and more. There was one memorable night in particular when I joined him on the porch as we let the rain fall on us. I don't recall if it was his idea or mine to join him, but it was just us two guys in the rain. It was like washing our worries and sins away to refresh for whatever lay ahead. It was a simple thing, but it meant something to me, and with Paco, it was the start of doing more things my age, because in more ways than one, he gave me the independence to do so. I was sixteen that summer, and I know most others my age weren't being forced to get in bed as early as 9:00 p.m. because their home nursing aide had arrived for nightly care. I hated how my day used to end just because my nurse arrived. And I hated when other people could not see past the physical disabilities and treat me with the same respect as any other teenager who by that age normally had a driver's license and/or a job and no forced bedtime. But when Paco came around, those things slowly began to change. We weren't going to parties, causing havoc, or whatever, but we did stuff like stay up for hours late into the night just talking about things or watching movies. One of the earliest memories was of us taking a walk after dark down to the Rt. 116 intersection just a quarter mile south of Rapatee. I finally felt like I was doing stuff my age instead of lying in home at bed. Nobody else my age was already in bed, so why should I be just because of my disabilities? That's just how I saw things. Around the same time frame of June, we sold the house in Rapatee and had a month to move out. As soon as I found out we were moving, with the help from the other kids, I had previously started packing up well ahead of time. Later, I was given a bit of grief for how poorly packed some of it was. I had a logical excuse; even though I had moved a lot, I never had much to pack when I was younger. Before I was burned, all my personal stuff could fit in one cardboard box. But now, I had a way lot more stuff than could fit in four to five boxes. Moving out of that house was a bittersweet moment for me. I was looking forward to a new place with more room and even a bigger yard so I could raise some more ducks again. But up to that point in my life, it was the longest I had stayed in any place. Even though it had only been three and a half years, it still seemed like much longer. One of the final things I remember doing was enjoying one last dip in the hot tub before we left. I honestly didn't want to join them because all I had were the clothes I was in and I didn't like the idea of my jeans and normal day clothes soaking wet. Not to mention it was almost exactly like a bath, and that meant the usual body cream Aquaphor and dressing treatment that came with a normal shower. Paco and Joey would *not* accept no for an answer, and so I ended up joining them after all.

We moved from Rapatee to a place in Maquon owned by a family friend of Vicki and Lee's. Her name was Sue, and when I first met her, she owned a bar in Maquon, but that year, she moved her bar to a bigger place in Elmwood. Moving went pretty quickly because we had a lot of helping hands, including the moving truck drivers. The house was not at all wheelchair friendly. The main entrance had two sets of stairs to enter the first floor, no bedrooms on the first floor, and both the bathroom and kitchen were tiny. Because of the odd room arrangements, I ended up sharing a room in the basement with Paco. Being in the basement actually didn't bother me much. The only disadvantage it had was not having my power chair available to me and not to mention the showers I had to endure down there, but I had no choice in either matter. Other than that, I loved that room down there. The basement was actually clean and in great livable condition. It was much bigger than my old room and stayed much cooler on hot days. Everyone knows growing teen boys need their sleep, and the lack of sunlight made it easier to sleep in longer during the day. Back then, neither Paco or me enjoyed getting up very early, but quite often, I had no choice because the home nurse aide had to come in to give me my shower every morning. But I almost always ended up going right back to sleep. But I also had to deal with the physical therapist showing up randomly, thus annoyingly disrupting my sleep. I didn't hate the therapists; I was just a teenager who didn't want to deal with that stuff, especially if it meant waking me up from deep slumber. Everything went smoothly moving into the new house, except for one little detail. As soon as we arrived and began getting stuff off the moving truck, my cat Max was put in my room to keep him safe and out of the way. But that plan didn't go well, and he almost immediately got outside and took off to roam the new place he was in. I was worried about him all day and hoped he would return safely. Whenever I was outside that day, I was roaming around the house, looking for him. That evening, I was still looking for him and quickly passed between Kyle and Michael, who were playing catch with a football. Kyle, being the jerk he occasionally was back then, decided to lob the ball at me after I had gone by. That's when Paco stepped in, and the inevitable fight ensued. It wasn't very physical, but it's almost inevitable with every foster kid who stayed with us long enough that eventually for whatever reason he'd get into a fight. We all got yelled at, including me, but I was just concerned and looking for Max. I wasn't bothering Kyle and Mike by quickly going between them. It wasn't as if they were playing hot potato and couldn't hold onto the football. Later on that night, Paco and I were just hanging out in our new room when I noticed movement in the window well, and I saw Max sitting there, staring and meowing at us. Paco quickly flipped open the window to let the confused cat in, and I was relieved he found his way back safely.

After camp, summer was mostly repetitive, with much of it spent in the basement just hanging out biding our time. Vicki and Lee's initial plan was to renovate the house where her small business was located and move in to that place. At first, I didn't like the idea because the house wasn't wheelchair friendly either. The house itself was smaller than the house in Rapatee, and with the plan to put my room in the converted garage, I would be cut off from the house because it was a different level than the rest of it. The garage was pretty large, and I liked that idea, but not after I learned the real plan was to split it and make each bedroom for two. The two main reasons I did like the idea of moving there were that I'd have a larger room with more space and the fact that there was already a chicken coop in the backyard where I could raise some ducks and/or chickens. But after I did find out the actual renovation plan, my whole acceptance of it changed. When I found out, I was already sharing a room with Kyle, and we tended to clash sometimes. Moving was supposed to better our living situation, not make it worse, and the plan to move to that little house outside Farmington was definitely not the best idea and definitely not worth leaving the old place in Rapatee. Summer dragged on, and my sister continued with her slow downward drop, making herself out to be a victim, but earlier that summer, around May or so, at the end of a supervised family visit in Galesburg, my sister and I were getting back in the car with our caseworker when Cassandra started to cry and didn't want to go. Back then, I firmly believed it was their fault for being in foster care. They had been out of control when they were still at home with my mom, and now, some of my siblings were having a difficult time adjusting to living in foster care. I don't recall exactly what I said, but my mom replied in not-so-exact words that it was my fault that she and my other siblings were in foster care. That obviously wasn't true, and initially, I was pissed off that she would say something like that. I got over it fairly quickly, but that little comment actually ended visits with my mom for a few years. I honestly thought the incident was used as an excuse for not taking me to the visits, but back then, all of my siblings had somewhat of a roller coaster relationship with my mom for a time. In the meantime, Paco and I continued to strengthen our friendship, and sometimes, we'd walk into town to the library or whatever we could find to do. Almost every day, Paco would put his Guns N' Roses tape in his very outdated Boombox and blast "Paradise City" and "Sweet Child O' Mine" as loud as he could even if Mystic stomped on the ceiling to make him turn it down. We would have played on my stereo, but Vicki was using it in her shop at the time. To this day, I can't play either song without thinking back to him and rocking out in that basement. With help from him and Peggy, who was increasingly helping out more during the evenings, the impact of the nightly visits from home health were kept to a minimum. As a result, many of our nights were spent just chatting away into the late morning hours about anything and everything. The more we bonded as summer went on, it suddenly dawned on me one day that his friendship had helped me move past my depression and my breakup with Amanda. And finally, I was doing things that made me feel more my age. Before I met Paco, it was as if I was missing out on a part of adolescence I wouldn't otherwise have gotten to experience. He helped me that summer in more ways than he knows, and he will always be a brother to me.

The only annoying part of the entire summer was disrupted sleep when the morning nurse would come in for my shower or my therapist showed up. At least I was getting more freedom in the evenings, but there was one particular day I remember when, for some reason, I just wasn't feeling good. Vicki's mom, Elaine, worked for Spoon River Home Health back then and stopped by to check me out. She still seemed to hold a grudge from our past bad experience, and she asked me if I didn't feel good. I replied by shaking my head no. Annoyingly she said, "What?" I shook my head no again, to which she once again said, "What?" albeit just a little bit louder than the first time. When I caught on the second time and answered no, she then said, "See, you can talk." Later, after Elaine had left, I mentioned to Vicki about her mom's rudeness. What harm was it when I answered her by shaking my head no? I wasn't feeling well, so she could have at least cut me a little slack, but then she had to utter those impolite words if only just to piss me off. The best part of that summer, aside from getting the new PlayStation and gradually becoming best friends with Paco, was finally being able to spend the night with Joey and the Spences' in Galesburg. Unfortunately, by the time I was finally able to spend the night, Elric was no longer living there. From what I heard, they simply grew tired of his lying, and thus, he ended up moving to a different home. Finally, staying overnight with Joey was yet another step toward more age-appropriate things that other teens my age were able to do—things like staying up late, going out all day to the mall or whatever, hanging out, etc. Not so much early on, but it was a big step up versus being forced to get in bed at 9:00 p.m. back home because my nurse had shown up. One of the first times I stayed with Joey was when I was invited to join the Spences on a trip to see a Bears-Packers training game up in Wisconsin. Back then, Christine and Joe did a lot of photography work, which included sports. Quite often, they could use their press access to get better seats of whatever event they might be at. We got up early, and unfortunately, when we arrived at the college where the game was to be, the rain put a damper on our plans. I don't remember if Joe didn't want to go because of the rain or the teams canceled, but our plans changed, and from there, we went to the famous House on the Rock. That place was so awesome. The only downside was not having my power chair. I hated being pushed around, but it also made some of the high places a bit tenser than I'd have been otherwise. For somebody who has never been there, the place is somewhat hard to explain. First of all, the place is huge, and it can take a few hours to walk through and see everything. I describe it as like a freakishly designed mansion/funhouse built directly on top of a cliff. You could say it's filled with a small village, and inside included things like automated music machines, antiques, and circus stuff. It really is hard to explain, and you have to see for yourself, but the two things I must point out is that it is home to the world's largest indoor carousel, and the end of the tour is the infinity room, which has 3,264 windows, extends 218 feet over valley, and 156 feet above the forest floor. Unfortunately, the infinity room is the only part inaccessible to wheelchairs because of a very narrow entrance. I'll say again that place was awesome and, in my honest opinion, worth the trip and worth missing the football game.

By the time midsummer had come around, my Bridgeway caseworker Samantha had left, and Pam had taken her place. Almost immediately, she had taken it upon herself to help me acquire a used van with a wheelchair lift. Vicki had the Ford Aerostar, but the constant lifting of me and my wheelchair was a strain on both of us, and it would only get more difficult as time passed. Having a van with a lift would be a leap forward toward furthering my independence in hopes that I could eventually equip it with the proper adaptive devices I'd need to safely drive it. There was no doubt about my physical ability to drive. I had already been examined at IPMR (Institute of Physical Medicine and Rehabilitation) to determine if I was capable of driving if I could acquire the necessary equipment. My reaction times were excellent, and all was good. I simply required the devices to drive. The next step would be an actual behind-the-wheel driving lesson. We were trying to get the school to pay for a behind-the-wheel session in Chicago, but in the meantime, we did our best to try to convince D.C.F.S. to pay for a van. When we learned that the uncle of Bobbi Jo was selling his van, Pam quickly jumped at the opportunity but first drove Paco and me to Canton to check it out. My first reaction was, "At least it wasn't a Chevy." Beggars couldn't be choosers, and for how much her uncle was asking for it, I thought it would be perfectly fine. I was given a test ride, and then we headed back home. So we had found a van but still needed to convince D.C.F.S. to provide the funding. It was easier said than done with constant pushing and pulling between the parties involved—Bridgeway, D.C.F.S., DHS, the van's owner, and of course, Vicki and me. But as with everything we usually did, the process was never easy, and they say good things come to those who wait. I was always waiting so long for many different things in life, so I still find it rather annoying when anyone dares say I have no patience. What I have no patience for is anyone telling me I have no patience!

In August, with just a week or two left until school started up again, Vicki and Lee took Paco, Cassandra, and me to the state fair in Springfield. The first thing different about it was the fact that Kyle and Mystic were off elsewhere, doing other things. Vicki almost never made random spur-of-the-moment stuff without usually including one of her own kids, but what was also unusual was Lee coming along. He came whenever we went to dinner or sometimes shopping but normally stayed home for most stuff like that. It was an easy road trip down to Springfield. Typically, somebody acted up on the drive there or back, and quite often, it was Kyle or Mystic. Usually, it was

Kyle who tended to start trouble just because he could. But when his victim spoke up because they grew tired of it, then automatically they are blamed too. For example, he might be punching me or whatever, and I speak up and become part of the problem. Why should I be forced to sit quietly and tolerate it? We weren't related by blood, but it was sibling rivalry at its worst. That was my first time visiting the state fair. I always saw the Heart of Illinois Fair in Peoria every year on TV and wanted to go to that one, but it was almost always too hot. Usually, the state fair was hot also, but we went later in the day than most would, especially considering how far we had to drive. We had dinner at a buffet before entering the fairgrounds, and then Paco and I just roamed around, mostly checking out the vendors. We both had a few bucks to spend, but as soon as he saw it, Paco just had to have a handmade poncho. Then not far from where he bought the poncho, we saw a novelty shirt mocking the famous three wise monkeys proverbial quote: "See no evil, hear no evil, speak no evil." But instead of three monkeys, this shirt had four, and the quote was changed to "See no sh———, hear no ———." You get the idea. And then the fourth was TAKE NO ———! We were laughing and thought it was worth buying, so we fought over it, and then both of us bought one. Before we left, I had just a few bucks left, but I wanted to buy a black leather wallet for $10. I was a little short, but Vicki told me to try haggling with the vendor selling it, but I was no good at haggling at all. I was a pushover. I gave up too fast and ended up paying the actual price. I simply wasn't comfortable with the whole haggling concept. You must be confident, not afraid of confrontation, nor willing to back down. Not to mention good hearing comes in handy too, but that I definitely lacked. That was probably my last favorite summer memory of just the two of us before school resumed.

Aside from the state fair, one of the last things we did before summer was over was we had to take a trip up to the Chicago suburb Wheaton. Somehow, we succeeded in getting the school to pay for a behind-the-wheel examination at Marianjoy Rehabilitation Hospital. Unlike the trip to the state fair, the van was fully loaded with six kids plus Vicki and Peggy, who by then was pretty much a full-time nanny. When she wasn't working her normal job, she was usually at our place helping out. The ride up there was long and boring as usual. But back then, we didn't have the convenience and luxury of today's fancy electronic gadgets like .mp3 players, mobile DVDs, and GPS, which now allow drivers to get to destinations as fast as possible. So our drive was longer than usual, mostly because for some reason Vicki took a long route off the interstate and toll ways when we were within the last seventy-five miles or so. When we finally arrived in Wheaton, we dropped most everyone else off at Target while Vicki and I went to my driving evaluation at Marianjoy. We then met Anne Hegberg, who was the head driver's rehabilitation specialist. Prior to my arrival, my appointment and the equipment were set up for driving a car. That's when we realized the school messed up. Anne told us the school had paid for a car evaluation and not a van. She agreed and insisted a car training session would not meet my physical needs and thus inappropriate for my disability. At first, Vicki and I were angry with the school and thought we had made the five-hour trip for no reason, but after a short evaluation and even though it wasn't paid for, Anne allowed me to take just a quick drive around the local facility in a properly equipped van. That first time driving, I was nervous and constantly worried my mirrors would hit something. But other than that, I was excited to finally learn that if I had the proper adaptive equipment, I was physically capable of driving a vehicle. After the short drive, I was also given a quick evaluation for a much-needed new wheelchair. So even though the school had messed up and I didn't get as much time behind the wheel as I would have liked, we did accomplish two things that day. First and foremost was the fact that given the right equipment, I could indeed drive. That knowledge alone was a huge confidence builder and gave me something to look forward to in my near future. Second was getting the ball rolling on acquiring a new wheelchair. We had tried prior to get a new wheelchair, but it had always been and still is a lengthy annoying process full of red tape. By then, my first wheelchair was already six years old and showing its age. It seemed like every summer it was out of commission for a month or two at a time because something internal had somehow gotten wet, usually from a water fight, I'd blow a tire, or I'd snap a drive belt because the slightest grain of sand tended to easily break them.

After the shortened driving evaluation, we picked up the others, and from there, we proceeded north on I-94 toward Gurnee and Six Flags. I knew we were in Scott Vaughn's neighborhood and tried but failed to get ahold of him while up there. When we got to Gurnee, there was still plenty of time to kill that day, so we all went to the Gurnee Mills mall. That place was huge, and at the time, it was the largest mall I'd ever been to. The only downside was not having any cash to spend every time I saw something I liked in yet another shop. I don't remember where we ate dinner, but we stayed at one of the more affordable hotels, and the plan for the next day was Six Flags. That night, Vicki was able to persuade me into getting into the hotel pool. As I've mentioned before, just sitting there is somewhat boring, no fun, and the water has a completely different feel to my skin. Not to mention that I was also kind of uncomfortable getting into a pool in public view. Doing so in front of my foster family and especially at camp didn't bother me at all, but unfamiliar, curious, and gawking eyes just made it that much more unappealing to me. In the pool, Vicki just kind of held me up while just sitting on the pool's underwater steps. I watched some girls tossing a beach ball around the other end, and everything was going fine as could be expected until the ball was hit and accidently landed very close to me. Personally, I was fine, but Vicki shouted at the girls something about me trying to safely enjoy my time in the pool. No harm, no foul. I knew it wasn't on purpose, and I didn't see anything wrong with what happened. I didn't want the special treatment because it just attracted more attention that I didn't want in the first place. To be honest, I find it difficult to explain how I feel about situations like that. The next day though, everyone was looking forward to spending the day at Six Flags. Most of us went our separate ways. Paco went off to explore the park on his own, and a few of us stayed with Vicki. For me, the first ride of the day was the Sky Trek Tower. Basically, you sit in an enclosed cabin, and it slowly rises to just over twenty-eight stories above the park. As it rises, it also rotates, which gives you a 360-degree view of the park. I don't like heights, but that one wasn't bad at all. Next, I remember being excited about a ride simulating a launch on the space shuttle. That kind of ride easily ranks among my favorite type. But when we got in the ride, attendants told Vicki I would be unable to sit in the motion seats and would just have to stay in my wheelchair for the ride. I was disappointed, of course, yet another example of missing out in life. Oh, it was awesome just being inside when the ride started, *but not really.* Without the effects of motion and movement, it was just a movie. I never had a problem at any previous park on a ride I wanted to go on. I don't remember what came next, but not much later, we went on to my favorite ride. At the St. Louis Park, it was called Thunder River, but the Chicago Park called it the Roaring Rapids. When we approached, the attendants once again told us I couldn't ride. By then, I was super annoyed and upset, as was Vicki. If I couldn't go on my favorite ride, then what was the point of being there? So Vicki and I went down to a service desk near the park entrance and told them about my problems with the rides and how I never had any such issues at the other park near St. Louis. After a short discussion, our tickets were refunded, and we were given vouchers for the St. Louis Park. So after getting our group back together, we headed back home. We were let down twice that trip, first at Marianjoy, but still gained something from that trip at least, unlike Six Flags, because we never did use the free tickets we got that day. Disappointment is inevitable in life, but at least I was satisfied going home with the knowledge that I could indeed drive. That alone was worth the entire trip and a huge morale boost in my hopes and plans for the future.

Chapter 29

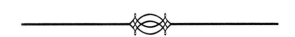

Before I knew it, summer was over, and I was back at Spoon River Valley High School to suffer through the various classes of the day. I was now a junior, and the biggest change that year was my new personal aide Joyce. Travis, the other disabled student at SRV, was now in the same building, and because of conflicting schedules, our aide Carl obviously couldn't be in two places at once. So Carl stayed with Travis, and Joyce was now my aide. Carl had a quiet personality, and I never really had a problem with him, other than perhaps the rare situations that I would have appreciated more privacy and discretion. Joyce, on the other hand, was very different. Instead of doing her job as described, which was helping me as needed, she also felt the need to order me around. I tried my best to shrug it off and ignore it for the most part, but what annoyed me most is when she would make me feel inferior. For example, sometimes when I'd ask her for something in front of other students, she would reply with a weird condescending look on her face, "What?" I never said anything about it, but I hated it so much. When she did that, it made me look like an idiot. She didn't look past my scars and disability to treat me like an equal human being. She treated the other students my age or younger with respect and interacted normally with them without the need to order them around, so why was I any different? Every day

I thought to myself, *You are here to help me out, not boss me around*, but I tolerated it till the very end. Probably my favorite class that year included being on the yearbook staff. Other than using a camera, I actually enjoyed the class quite a bit. The class was one of many I had with Mrs. Suter while at Valley, and even though we tended to give her a hard time, sometimes she was still one of the "cooler" teachers, and I tended to do well in her classes. Over the course of the year, we went on at least two field trips just for the yearbook. The first one was in Macomb at Western Illinois University. That was actually my first time seeing WIU, and we were there to attend a kind of lecture for tips on making a great yearbook. The guy speaking was a representative from Jostens, and initially, when he tried to get the students to participate, obviously the room was quiet enough to hear a pin drop. When somebody was finally brave enough to say something, he awarded them with a $100 bill. When he asked another question, pretty much every hand in the room shot up as fast as possible. I guess that's one way to motivate people. The other trip was later on in the second half of the school year, because I know it was during the first Teenie Beanie Baby craze at McDonald's. We went to Canton and basically went around town, trying to sell ads in our yearbook. Without money from the ads, we simply couldn't afford it otherwise. For lunch, we went to McDonald's, and surprisingly, Joyce bought two full Happy Meals for herself. Obviously, she wanted the beanies, but in the process, she had spilled my drink. Logic and kindness dictated that she might share one of her drinks with me, but nope, that didn't happen.

At home, around the same time that school had begun, I started going to CIL (Center for Independent Living) in Peoria for various things, like assertiveness training, disabled rights, and computer club. It started with the assertiveness training and slowly branched out from there. Initially, that was how Vicki and I gradually learned that as my time in high school was winding down, there were things the school was required to provide but wasn't. For example, the behind-the-wheel training was one of those. The school had given in to that, probably hoping and thinking it would be enough to push it aside, and for the time being, it was fine, except for when the faculty and everyone else involved came together for my IEP (Individualized Education Plan) sessions. In Vicki's words, "The meetings at the IEP's were always a battle. They always tried to get by without meeting your needs. Some of the issues were things like driver's ed. They said we had to buy a van and equip it for you before they would send you to Chicago to learn to drive. I told them that they couldn't make us do that. No other kid in the United States had to buy a vehicle before they were given driver's ed. So they couldn't hold us to any other standards either." I was already at school for eight hours a day, so I never wanted to spend a minute longer, but even though it was always extremely boring, they were very necessary in terms of asserting my rights as a student with physical disabilities. As the years progressed, more people became involved with my IEP. There was the school administration, my teachers, physical therapist, my foster care social worker Pam, my CIL advisor Holly, my lawyer whom we hired after the bullying incidents, and John Miller from CIL, who was deaf and an advocate for my hearing issues. The IEP sessions could get pretty heated sometimes. During one session when John Miller was present, his sign language interpreter had momentarily stopped signing. From what I learned later on, a signer is paid and required to translate everything during the session. That included conversations between two people. The interpreter would stop to talk or not catch everything, and John became upset. He tried to tell her she needed to be signing for him, but it also became apparent that she couldn't read sign language. John was angry and understandably frustrated while the interpreter also seemed obviously uncomfortable. It was the school's responsibility to provide a sign language translator, and she couldn't even read what she signed to do her job properly. It was just another example of the school trying to do the bare minimum.

Around late September, Paco finally moved out after repeated delays. All summer, he was constantly told he'd be moving out only to be turned back again. I was glad he stuck around as long as he did, but I was very confident that his time with us wasn't forever and that he would indeed eventually move out. I enjoyed our time together hanging out, and over the summer, we had become brothers. I was happy for him that he was able to move in with his brother and be with his family, though I can honestly say I was still sad to see him go. But life goes on, and true friendships will always remain strong. He said his good-byes, and off he went to live with his brother Juan in Galesburg. After Paco moved out, Kyle moved in, and that's when I started to have serious doubts and apprehension about the prospect of us sharing a room in the new house. For whatever reason, Kyle and I just seemed to clash sometimes; typically, it was something he did. Even though I was older, he did what he wanted with even my stuff, but he also had a double standard. One night, he listened to a CD all night on my stereo without shutting it off. I couldn't sleep at all, and when Vicki told him to leave it off the next night, he complained. Or another example would be forcing me to pause or stop a movie while he was occupied, and yet if I asked him to do the same for me, it wasn't happening. Kyle could be just fine sometimes, but occasionally, his logic just threw me off, as if his rights and comforts were more important than mine. There was one time when we were in the van and I was seriously overheating because he had the AC vents shut. Vicki told him to open them, but he said, "He was cold." Or the night I wanted to watch a new episode of *Star Trek: Voyager* on my own TV in our shared room, he yelled and fought with Vicki about it. He liked the show too, but because he had already seen the episode, he didn't care and wanted to shut it off. If the situation was reversed, it would have been just fine. Go figure. So I don't remember exactly when it was decided, but eventually Vicki and Lee came to an agreement that instead of renovating and moving into the rental house near Farmington, we should build a new house best suited for everyone. My seventeenth birthday was somewhat simple without too much glamour as the past few years had been sometimes. I got a few new movies for my VCR because my poor TV had no channel reception in the basement at all. That left me with three options for entertainment—my stereo, VCR, or my PlayStation. If I did want to watch a show, I had to go upstairs, but the living room TV still lacked the closed captioning I needed. But my favorite birthday gift that year was the original *Need for Speed* PlayStation game that Bob and Diane gave me. Until then, my previous games all summer were the demos and Shockwave Assault, which was actually a dud. But NFS was an awesome racing game, which in my opinion blew all previous racing games away and set the stage for other racing games in the future. Not only were the graphics and everything so far from previous game systems, but it included actual video about each car in the game. I quickly became adept at it, and back then, even Kyle couldn't beat me, though he would probably still deny it.

After my birthday, there was so much going on at the time that I can only guess what was going on at any specific time. The first IEP was usually around this time, Spoon River Drive, winter approaching, holidays, etc. and all the other stuff thrown into the mix that was happening simultaneously. Sometime before Thanksgiving, I headed back down to Shriners in Galveston for more reconstructive surgery. By then, it had been a year and half since my previous surgery, so the time had come again to face the knife, so to speak. Before my surgery, I had to have a central line IV put in. That alone was basically surgery because I had to be given anesthesia for the procedure. What's funny is, when I woke up in the recovery room that particular time, I was unusually happy. I wasn't "high" happy. I guess I was happy because it went fast and smooth, and I was still a lot more comfortable than

I would be if I had just underwent an actual reconstructive surgery. As usual, my eyes were blurred and couldn't see or focus at all, but the recovery room technician that particular day seemed nicer, and with how comfortable and positive I was feeling in the moment, we actually had a nice conversation. And even though I can't remember what we talked about, I do remember having a song stuck in my head and just kind of tapping my leg on the bed while playing it over and over in my head. Ironically, it wasn't even a Bon Jovi song. For some random reason, I had Michael Jackson's "Beat It" song stuck in my head. I really can't explain why my experience in the recovery room that day had such an effect on me, except for the fact that I wasn't burdened with the miserable side effects of an actual painful surgery. It wasn't all rainbows and unicorns, though, to be honest. Later that evening, when I was trying to watch *Star Trek: Voyager*, I was feeling a little uncomfortable from the anesthesia while Vicki was out getting dinner. She was always there when I came back to my room, and it helped me so much to know she was there for me when I needed it most, but eventually, everyone must eat, and sometimes that's when I needed her. After the central line had been put in, Vicki and I bided our time until the actual surgery. I had an open sore on my back, and they wanted it to heal a little bit before my surgery. What I couldn't help but wonder was the fact that I had numerous sores in the past during surgeries, so why would it be such a big deal now? As we waited, we also eventually found out that my surgeon Dr. McCauley had supposedly gone to New Orleans and wouldn't be back soon. Frustrated and irritated, we let the hospital staff know that I couldn't sit there idly waiting for him to come back. Every day in the hospital was another day I missed school, and I simply couldn't afford the cost at the time. Even if I waited till he returned, I still had an extended healing time which further increased the duration of my stay. I was annoyed because my time had been wasted and both Vicki and I kind of felt as if I were a guinea pig or personal project. This is a small part of Vicki's experience at my side in the hospital, in her words "Major was surgery very painful, but we had been there for 2 weeks or more and he hadn't done the surgery. We had just been waiting around and nothing was being done. If my memory serves me correctly I asked Gene if your surgery was even scheduled yet. I was told NO, that your doctor was out of town for another week and a half. I then told Gene that I was going to make arrangements and I was taking you home. So he called McCauley and put us on the phone together. He told me he didn't need me there to do the surgery and I could go home. I informed him that I did need to be there for you. I always worried about you after surgery because not all the nurses were that great to you. So I always wanted to be with you and stay after surgery till I knew you could fend for yourself. It was Major surgery and that nobody should have to go through that alone. It really upset me. So I said to him this may your ball field that we are playing ball in but Caper is your star player and we are not waiting around in this hospital any longer. We are leaving tomorrow. He told me we couldn't do that. I told him I felt we had been sitting there waiting for him to decide and do the surgery long enough. I was taking you back home and back to school. And when he was ready to operate give us a call. I do remember in 1993 when you had your axillas done I reported a nurse for being less then professional with you. And that is why I always felt I needed to be there for you. It was on a Thursday morning and the doctors were making grand rounds and when doctors made grand rounds the nurses were supposed to have their patients ready for the doctors. That meant to have all dressings and casts off of the patients so the doctors didn't have to wait around. Anyway I remember this today like it was yesterday, you were only a few days post op. and because she had put off getting you ready she didn't have time to give you any pain medicine. She came in and jerked off your splints and you started Crying. And then she said to you "knock off that crying and quit being such a big Baby". I was shocked and heartbroken and it was all I could do to hold back my tears. When the doctors came in the room Dr. Herndon said "Caper what's wrong', you told him you were in a lot of pain. So they ordered X-rays of your Shoulders they thought maybe they had accidentally broken them when they were manipulating the arms/armpits for the skin grafts. Little did they know it was caused by a nurse. I didn't say a thing. About an hour later Catherine came by your room. She took one look at me and asked me what was wrong! I started to cry and told her what had happened she told me I needed to report the nurse for what she had said and done. Later that day I was sent to see Pat Blakeney and then was sent to head of nursing to tell them what had happened. I told them if this happened with me standing right there what would that nurse be capable of doing or saying without me there. That's a scary thought" I was always grateful Vicki was there with me after surgery. And what she said is a big reason for it. Not only was I helpless after surgeries but I couldn't fend for myself either, which is a huge part of why the surgeries of summer 1991 were so difficult. I went through that entire summer alone, without an advocate, and nobody in my room at my side to help me when I needed it most. I was surprised to actually see Vicki cry over all that was going on, and that showed me how much it truly affected her. One of the hospital social workers asked me how I could dare stand up to Dr. McCauley. To be honest, I do respect and appreciate what he does, but like most doctors, I still found him intimidating, but I replied truthfully and honestly in almost these exact words: "I am missing school, and I don't have time to sit here and do nothing," so after two weeks in a hospital room waiting and with nothing accomplished, we gave up and went back home.

The only positive thing from not having surgery done while I was in Galveston was the fact my hair was able to stick around that much longer. I had been growing my hair for over a year with almost no cutting, and I was trying to grow it out a bit. In previous years, every time it had grown out, I was given a cut to trim my bangs. The trimming effectively held back any progress I made toward growing it out. When I realized my progress was purposely being inhibited, I said enough was enough and was finally able to start growing my hair out the way I wanted. There were a few different reasons I had wanted longer hair. First off was sort of homage to Bon Jovi. Second, the longer hair helped to cover the sides of my head where hair could not grow. Third, growing my hair was kind of my way of rebelling. Paco looked great with his long hair, so why couldn't I? Lots of people put stereotypes on long hair and label them as troublemakers. But a person's hair doesn't determine who they are. Take the time to get to know the person inside, and you might be surprised. In Paco's case, I know I was surprised, and I'm glad I took the time to get to know him.

Almost immediately after getting back home, it seemed like we were moving again. The plan with the new house was to build on some land just west of London Mills on Rt. 116. So in order for us to be closer during the building process, we moved from Maquon into an older house where they had lived in years before they lived in Rapatee. I was happy that progress was being made toward a new house and the fact that Paco was helping us move that weekend. Even though we had almost no time to talk or hang out, it was still good to see him since he moved out a month or two before then. It was an older house on a hill just north of London Mills and about the same distance from school as the previous place in Maquon. To be honest, the house wasn't much better than the one before. They both had their own positives and negatives. I still shared an even smaller room with Kyle, but at least I had some reception on my tiny TV. But probably the biggest annoyance was the inconvenience of my daily shower. Every morning, the ritual began with me being pushed out of my room through the living room and kitchen to the bathroom. The shower itself wasn't pleasant, because it was a much-older-style bathtub, which made me feel more exposed, and not to mention *cold*, while being given my shower. I also hated seeing myself in the mirror which faced the bathtub. Honestly, who wants to watch themselves bathe? And then there was the makeshift ramp I had to face every morning when I left for school. The ramp itself was just two wooden planks. It wasn't very high, but it didn't need to be for me to still get hurt if I were unfortunate enough to drive off the side. Luckily for me, it never did happen. Almost simultaneously with moving, I think the very first following Monday back to school the brand-new wheelchair-lift-equipped school bus was finally ready. That for me was an experience I had left behind since my days riding the school bus from Douglas to Yates City. Even though I rode a bus when I went to school in Peoria, most of the time, I was the only rider. I was reminded how boring riding a school bus with dozens of kids can be and waiting your turn to finally be dropped off. I wasn't looking forward to riding with a new group of kids whom I had not yet met, who had to be wondering just who the heck I was and where I suddenly came from. The students from the junior and senior high school building obviously knew who I was, but most of the elementary students had yet to see me face-to-face. The first morning, all went smoothly on the ride to school, with a few curious glances my way. The ride home, on the other hand, didn't go so well. In the morning, a different bus didn't pick up the preschoolers until noon or so but then rode the same bus back home with everyone else. Travis and I were already on the bus before everyone else, followed by the elementary students, then the junior and senior high school students. The drama started when one of the preschoolers got on the bus and freaked out as he went to his seat. The poor boy was crying, and I remember a girl just a few years older trying to comfort him, but it didn't help him much. At that moment, I felt terrible, because I was obviously the source of his fear and there was nothing I could do. I never liked attracting attention to myself, and that kind of negative attention on that first day riding the bus was not helping anything. One boy stood out in particular as being most afraid, and I'm sure there were a few others, but it was at least a few days until any effort was made by the school to alleviate the fears of these kids. Vicki told me one boy supposedly brought a spray bottle to use as "monster spray." Finally, the mother of the boy most afraid of me brought him and his sister to our house to meet me and show I was a person just like them and they had nothing to be afraid of. She was one of my nurses with Spoon River Home Health and so was able to set up a time to introduce her kids to me outside school and in her presence, with encouragement and a parental figure nearby to reassure them. Both kids actually got past their fears pretty quickly when they saw that despite my physical appearance I was still a person just like them. I had my interests, hobbies, needs, music, etc. just like any other person, and that helped them push aside the fears of my scars to no longer see a monster but instead a human being with needs whom their own mom helped care for.

I think it was sometime around early December when I got my first call for a job interview. I had recently watched the news and found out that Target was doing its best to hire employees with disabilities. I figured it wouldn't hurt to apply, and I was surprised when I got the call a few days later while I was staying with Bob and Diane one weekend. Vicki took me in for the interview the following Monday, and I admit I didn't really know what to expect. Vicki also sat in for the interview, but prior to then, I had not yet taken any classes involving job applications and/or interviews, though ironically just a few months later during one of my second semester classes, it came up in my junior achievement class. Vicki was there sort of as advisor/support/translator role even though I did have my hearing aid, but to put it bluntly, bringing along a parent/guardian or pretty much anyone with you to an interview was bad interview etiquette. But one thing I remember is they asked me at least one question I now know they couldn't legally ask, and that was about my transportation. Vicki answered that one for me, and in her own way and said, "It's taken care of." To be honest, I didn't know what I would be physically capable of and what things my particular job might be required of me. But in the end, I received a call and was told simply, "We aren't really hiring right now." I knew this obviously wasn't true, because all major retailers were adding more employees for the holiday rush. Very rarely does anyone ever get the job after their first interview, so I actually wasn't surprised to be turned down. I didn't let it bother me at all and just wrote it off as a new experience and lesson learned. There's a first for everything in life, and I marked that one off my list.

A week or two before Christmas on the same day, we went to the Young Messiah Christmas concert we finally got the used van D.C.F.S. agreed to pay for. From the moment, we asked them there were a lot of red tape and pushing and pulling from all sides. We were actually optimistic that they might fund the van without much refusal. But the trouble came from all sides. At one point, the seller no longer wanted to sell us the van, which left us back at square one. But eventually, they agreed, and it took all those months in between to get everything straightened out and the van paid for. I was excited for the van because it meant no more tedious lifting in and out of the current van and I no longer had to rely on being pushed around in my manual wheelchair whenever we went somewhere. The freedom of mobility when out shopping was a huge change from relying on others to constantly push me around. Already, on that first night, we went to the aforementioned concert at the high school. But that was the one place where I already used my power chair on a daily basis. When we got inside, I was holding onto the keys, and I remember as I went past Darren, I said, "I got a new van." The van was another step toward independence and preparing me for later years. Almost immediately after getting the van, we found out there was a huge fine if we didn't get tie downs for my wheelchair. Surprisingly for some reason, none were previously installed, so we were forced to do so quickly. We took it to a place in Peoria and had them installed, and initially, I had hoped to eventually equip it so that I would be able to drive it myself. But after a few months had passed and we had a chance to take it up to Freedom driving aides in Chicago, we realized it wouldn't be worth the cost because the van was already aging. The adaptive equipment required was too expensive, so there was little point in spending so much on something that wouldn't last long term without problems. So for the time being, I was at least grateful I had a van with a lift and kept my hopes up for another van in the future that I could drive myself. That van basically was the best part of Christmas that year, aside from the Young Messiah concert at school. Usually, there was just the grade school kids singing the classics, but that year a separate performance was done, and it was amazing. That concert and the following year's performance are probably my fondest during the four years I attended. SRVHS was a small school with a smaller budget than most, but that show was well done and presented as if it were shown by a school with a much higher budget for extra-curricular activities. It helped make up for what was in my opinion a pitiful Christmas at home that year. We had gifts and the dinners, but because of moving and the fact that everything was in storage, Vicki had decided on no tree or decorations that year. She tried to assure me that we would get a huge tree the next year and go all out after we moved into the new house. A tree wasn't just somewhere to hang shiny ornaments and put presents under; it was a tradition that's been part of every Christmas since I was born. And I do know it's Christ's holiday, but a tree is part of those cherished childhood memories, and without the tree, part of that youthful magic of the season just isn't there. The past few years, I had stayed at home for Christmas, but I changed things up that year, and I spent the holiday with Bob and Diane. And even though they had an artificial Christmas tree, at least they had one, and they had lights up as well.

Chapter 30

The situation with my sister continued on a steady downhill drop. There was always something going on with her, and she was almost constantly in trouble for something. At one point, Vicki gave her an ultimatum and told her if she moved out, then I would be forced to move too. This was actually a bluff to get her to straighten up and fly right, because she knew that I was content to stay where I was. But I, on the other hand, knew she either would not care and/or was smart enough to realize that it in fact was a bluff on Vicki's part. I wanted her to get her act together, but I honestly didn't think it was going to happen. At least not while living with us and perhaps not any other foster home either. Even after Vicki made up a story and told Cassandra that I was crying one night because I was afraid of moving out her words and actions showed me she didn't really care. Classes at school during the remainder of my junior year in high school actually weren't too bad. The yearbook class continued, and it felt somewhat fulfilling to contribute to something and feel useful. I need help with many things, but it's nice when I can give back and be an active physical part of something no matter how small a part it may be. That part was the simple task of folding and stapling school newsletters to be mailed out. Then there was also my junior achievement class. Basically, it was a business class and included stuff like economics, marketing, résumés, and job interviews. About once a week or so, our teacher would ask us to write a little something about whatever product he brought up that day and how we would market it and so on. And the class also included field trips to the Peoria Regional Airport, where we saw how things operated at the mail processing facility and a bank in Canton which got our class mentioned in the Canton newspaper with a small article and a photo. I'm not sure if it was for the Junior Achievement course or my FFA class the following year, but we also took a field trip to the John Deere Distribution Center in Milan, Illinois. The trip also included a stop at the John Deere Pavilion downtown Moline. But the distribution center itself was interesting because the place was so huge. Much of it was automated to increase efficiency and delivery times, and it was cool to see how it all came together. Strangely enough, one of the things I remember standing out about that year and especially that particular semester were the trends within pop culture. During the holidays, that annoying red doll, which when you squeezed its belly said, "Ha ha, that tickles." Yes, I'm talking about the famous Tickle Me Elmo. Parents had gone insane for the toy, and finding one was like winning the lottery. I remember a girl bringing one to class. I didn't judge, but in my mind, I was like, *Seriously, was this high school or preschool?* But it didn't end there; even more popular but more affordable was the Beanie Baby craze. Heck, even I had one of those, but mine was given to me the previous summer at camp, months before most people were made aware that they existed. One huge difference between the Beanies and Elmo was that there were a lot of different beanies to choose from and the fact that people of literally all ages were snatching up Beanie Babies. Not only did I see grade school kids with Beanies pretty much every day, but even the high school students joined in the Beanie Baby insanity. I'll be honest, even though I already had one, I acquired one more when I saw a bag full of them Vicki had bought while in Canton. I innocently assumed she had bought one for everyone, and I saw the Leopard and claimed him. Oh no, I had given into pop culture and followed the crowd, but at least I didn't take it to school like everyone else did. Or did I?

Behind the scenes at school, my boring annual IEP sessions continued. But as mentioned earlier, we now had a lawyer present to try to keep the school in check. Even though the need for a lawyer began with the bullying and teasing situation, it soon escalated into much more than that. As time had passed, I increasingly got the feeling that things were going to get tense the closer I got to my graduation the next year. I had no doubts, and my grades were fine, but questions were raised whether or not I should aim for graduating on time. Every session was rushed and involved bickering between those involved. Some of the school administrators may have said whatever I needed they would take care of it, but I wasn't stupid. If that was indeed the case, then I wouldn't have needed a lawyer and my high school experience would have been a better one. All that and the fact that certain advisers were telling Vicki, my lawyer, and me that by law there were things the school still had to do but were not doing and the school basically hoped I'd graduate before they were forced to and thus no longer required to provide. After one particular session, Vicki noticed my lawyer talking to the principal alone. Afterward, she asked him what it was about, and he rudely told her he didn't have to tell her anything and that he only had to answer to me. Vicki said that she was my guardian and thus could speak for me in my best interests. Needless to say, after that little incident, he was gone, and we never did find out what was discussed between the two. Loyalty means a lot to me, and I despise backstabbers.

Aside from school matters, there was also plenty going on at home. Construction on the new house was slowly progressing, and both Vicki and Lee were constantly going back and forth, helping when they could. I was constantly asking when we'd finally move in, and time dragged on slowly. It seemed like forever since we had packed up our stuff for moving. And as time wore on, I increasingly hated sharing a room with Kyle. When you tend to butt heads with your roommate, afterward, there is nowhere to retreat to, no private sanctuary to call your own. That spring was typical in London Mills. It brought heavy rain, and that always meant flooding. I remember NBC WEEK 25 out of Peoria was covering the flood, and it showed a clip of Vicki driving through the floodwaters toward home. When that was recorded, the water was still low enough for her van, but it was deeper when our school bus headed home. I kept thinking. *She's not going to go through it, is she?* Driving around would take longer, but the safety of young riders is more important, you'd think. Personally, I would have gone around, but she slowly drove through it, and we made it home just fine. Still, we could have been in trouble if we hit something submerged or whatever, and these days, drivers are constantly bombarded with warnings not to drive through floodwaters and about how little water is needed before it can overtake your vehicle. By April, my spring fever is usually setting in, and I'm ready to spend more time outdoors. But there was one night when Vicki and Peggy came in and unplugged my computer, and I asked them, "What are you doing?" They said, "Remember when you said you wouldn't mind one more snowstorm? Well, you got your wish." I was only happy because it meant a day off from school, but a minute or two after they left my room, I heard a zap and the smell of smoke. At first, I thought Max had knocked over my computer, but actually an electrical surge had fried my surge protector. I had never seen an electrical surge or short, and I was at least grateful it wasn't anything worse.

I was also still going to CIL in Peoria for the computer group and independent living assertiveness, etc. It was also in April that I went on a trip by myself for the first time. I had a personal attendant provided by CIL to help me with my care, but other than that, I was on my own in a new place. The trip itself was to attend a three-day convention/seminar for people with disabilities. I was somewhat looking forward to going, and at least I was missing school, but I was nervous about the whole attendant situation because it was my job to show her every step of my daily morning care. Basically, it was the same situation as my very first camp, but instead of a group of counselors, only one person would help me with the majority of my needs. The day we left, I met up in Peoria with a few other people, including a few from my computer group. Most of us rode in the same van on the way down there. That was the first time I attended an event with such a large number of people in a convention-type setting. I'm always a little quiet with new people and large crowds, but the fact that we were all there because of our disabilities gave us a common bond and helped ease my nervousness. I had my own hotel room, and I couldn't help but feel like a celebrity in a posh suite. I'd spent the night in hotels before, mostly for stays outside the hospital in Galveston, but never for a convention/seminar. It had a totally different feel to it, as if I were a VIP and my reason for attending was important and beneficial not just to me but others I *associated* with. It's almost hard to describe attending such events, but I come from a low-income family, and every time I have had an opportunity to go, I can't help but feel so far from the world I was born into. The closest I can describe is like suddenly being famous. After all, celebrities are an exclusive group, and few are lucky to make it. The similarity isn't too far different from being disabled; we too are a select group, but for a different reason. Occasionally, a celebrity comes from a poor background and is thrust into money, fame, and luxury, a far cry from being poor. That's kind of how I'm trying to convey what it's like for me. It's not about the money, luxury, food, material things, etc., just the fact that it's so different from the social class that I come from. I did enjoy the event, and it's also healthy to experience new things and enlighten oneself. There's a big world waiting out there to be experienced and new people and cultures to meet. After the awkward first day with my attendant, things went smoother from then on, and I even became friends with her daughter Jasmine. I only wish we had kept in contact, but those were the days before Facebook and networking made such things so easy. Other than that, I don't remember any real detail, except for the closing ceremony dance on the final night. I was a little overheated that evening and decided to step outside for a few minutes of cooler fresh air. As soon as I was outside the door, I was just blasted by the wind. I like windy weather, but this was too much for even me, and I was just getting battered back and forth in my wheelchair. So back inside I went and eventually to my room, where I saw on the local station that there were tornado warnings and watches in the area. Springfield managed to avoid the severe stuff, but the same weather system had hit back home too. When I arrived home next day, the power was out, and the roads were blocked near Middle Grove, just east of the high school because an F1 tornado did some minor damage there. Later on, I even heard that they still allowed the students to board the buses despite that tornado being only two to three miles east. Stupid on their part, obviously, but I always seemed to be away from home when anything exciting happened.

After being open for almost a year or so, Vicki and Lee decided to close up the Old Oak Tree that spring. I guess it simply didn't earn enough profit, and afterward, Vicki and Lee simply sold that house, most likely to help pay for the new one. Before I knew it, the end of May had arrived, and that meant the end of the school year and my last summer break before I began my final year of high school when it resumed in the fall. The last day of school was the same as the previous year and just as pointless. A waste of money, bus fuel, lost sleep, and time missed out on video games and other summer break activities. I obviously didn't care to go but was hardly surprised when Vicki made us go anyway. She, of course, still had to work and I'm sure wanted to savor every last second she possibly could till school was officially over. Typically, there was at least one food fight near the end of the year as well as water fights on the buses during the ride home. The water fights weren't really allowed, but there was little to stop them from doing it anyway other than confiscating water guns and water balloons. It was the last day, so what punishment could anyone get other than that? For that same reason, I decided to push the boundaries a little bit, and I wore my "Monkey see no sh——, monkey take no sh——" profanity-laced shirt as my way of rebelling against authority, particularly school authority. I was nervous, but to my surprise, nobody said a word about it, not even Joyce. I was certain she would say something and chastise me or whatever, but nothing came of it. The day was just a quick in and out. I pretty much got off the bus, received my report card, lingered for a few pointless minutes, and then I was back on the bus and headed home by 10:00 a.m. or so. It was just a waste of time for something that could be mailed. When I got back home, summer had officially begun, camp was already on my mind, and with my junior year behind me, I looked forward to finishing my senior year at high school when it resumed in August.

Chapter 31

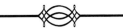

On the weekend we went to camp, Joey and I continued our tradition of me staying the night with him and the Spences' then going out for breakfast before heading to the fire station and off to camp. Other than that, camp '97 was a big change in comparison to the previous four years I had spent as a camper. I had my power wheelchair with me again that year, and even though I had it the previous year, the freedom of having it at camp still seemed fresh and new. But the biggest and most obvious difference was the simple fact that I was no longer a camper. I was a CIT (counselor in training). The CIT program was implemented to allow former campers to return to camp and volunteer as future counselors. The program included two and, when necessary, sometimes three years of training as a CIT. After those two to three years is junior counselor, which is pretty much just a title until full counselor is granted at age twenty-one. Though to be honest, there's little difference between junior counselor and full counselor. They both have the same responsibilities, but a full counselor simply has more experience. Back in those early years of the CIT program, it was much different than it is now, because they were learning as they went along. Also, keep in mind that not only did the CIT program evolve and change over the following years, but those changes also included different CIT staff that came and went. Different staff meant different ways of doing things. Over the years, there were always new faces to meet and bond with. Because it was still the easiest option in terms of my daily care and needs, Mike Kilburg and Scott Vaughn were still my counselors that year. Like I mentioned above, the CIT program was new to all of us, not just the CITs. I had friendships with so many at camp, and not just counselors but obviously my peers too. But naturally, we all tend to gravitate toward certain people in our lives, and some people stick out more than others. For example, I met Mara in '95, and in 97 was when I met Chelsea Leahy. She was one of the CDY staff counselors in unit 3, and as the week progressed, we got to know each other. She was only four years older than me, so when I talked to her, I felt more like an equal peer instead of a camper. But then again, a lot of the staff seemed to connect that way with me. They gave me the same dignity and respect as anyone they would fellow staff or other teens my age. Sometimes people just can't see past my scars and albeit small size and realize that, yes, in fact I'm much older than they think. Over the years, I've inspired so many to look at life, appreciate it, and enjoy it as I do. I truly feel great when friends and family tell me how I've inspired or helped them see their own lives in a more positive light. It gives me a sense of purpose and fulfillment, as if it's what I'm here to do. No matter what, there's always something to be grateful for even in the darkest moments. And if you let them in, there is always somebody who is willing to fight for you, stand with you, and be a shoulder to lean on.

Here is a little something from Chelsea Leahy about her first summer at camp: "The summer of 1997 was the year that I met Caper Brown. I was working at YMCA Camp Duncan through the International Camp Counselor Program, and the first camp for the summer was the IFSA Burn Camp. I was assigned to the senior group in the unit 3 area. I remember seeing Caper, who was also with the senior group, and wondering what his story was. All the kids had a story. I connected with Joey, Caper's younger brother, almost immediately, and through him I got to know Caper.

"I didn't hear what happened to Caper straight away; it was something that was spoken about in small increments. I don't really think I completely understood all that he endured until much later in our friendship. That one week that we spent together would change my life. I started looking at things with a whole different perspective. What Caper had achieved and overcome in his short seventeen years was unbelievable. Something like 113 surgeries. His zest for life was inspiring. He was such a great role model to all the new campers. If Caper could do it, then so could they.

"As the week was coming to an end, we had a camp disco. Caper had a plan! He was going to walk on his prosthetic legs in front of everyone. It was such an achievement for him and an amazing moment for everyone who had been a part of his recovery. All those that had watched him grow into the wonderful young man he now was.

"The last day was emotionally draining. I was a mess. I was sad that such a great week was over and sad that I was saying good-bye to my new friends. Something in my heart told me that I would see him again and that we would keep in touch. Caper and Joey were a huge part of me returning to camp for the summers of 1998, 1999, and 2000. It was so great to reconnect each year."

The actual CIT program that year mostly seemed to focus on the behind-the-scenes camp operations. We did a lot of helping out with the quartermasters with setting stuff up, snack times, cleanup, etc. Even though most of it seemed to be actual physical work, we still had opportunities to interact with the campers too. And just like the counselors, we were also given a night off, albeit as one large group. We went out for dinner, and I typically had a steak. Then we saw a movie before returning to camp that evening. Those CIT nights off were always one of the highlights of the week. It allowed us time to have fun, hang out, and enjoy each other's company without worrying about any camp schedules, campers, responsibilities, etc. It was IFSA's way of saying "Thank you for volunteering your week"

278

and a reminder how each and every individual is important to camp, and all are appreciated for what they do. As former IFSA director Mary Werderitch often says, "Volunteers aren't paid because they are worthless, but because they are priceless!" All of it just further motivation to return to camp in the future.

Sadly, I must mention it was late '96 when Nathan Boston passed away after returning home from a surgery. We held a tree dedication ceremony at camp in his honor. It has a permanent plaque that reads, "In loving memory, Nathan Boston. Burn Survivor, IFSA Burn Camp 1996." The dedication cast a different mood over everyone at camp. As far as I remember, it was the first time a former camper had passed away, and he was still so young. But it was especially difficult when his younger brother Jonathan was asked if he wanted to say anything. I completely sympathized with him, and it was painful to watch him as he broke down crying, unable to say anything because his loss was still too fresh and the pain too much. I'll never forget it as was one of the most emotional moments everyone at camp shared as a whole. I then thought of my relationship with my own brother and how terrible it would be to lose him. And then I felt bad because I thought I was being selfish by thinking of my own brother and "what if" instead of mourning Nathan and Jonathan's pain. I told Joey I wanted to die first when we grew old, but then he also said the same thing, so obviously, our feelings were mutual. After the dedication, we had a break period, and the majority of the campers and staff took the time to lie down, rest, and reflect on the ceremony. It was all we could do to unload after the overwhelming emotions that day. Even today, as time passes by day by day, that moment at camp was one of the earliest reminders of my own mortality. I don't like to think about the subject. Some people say I've already beaten the odds by far, but I want to continue to do so for a long time to come. I have a survivor mentality, and there's just so much I want to do, see, and be part of.

I had received a new pair of prosthetic legs earlier that year, and I got a nice new expensive pair of Nike's to go with them. I wanted a new look with that pair, so I asked that the outer leg appearance be left bare to show the inner steel skeleton of the prosthetic itself. I saw in pictures that a lot of amputees had their own prosthetics with this bare look, and I thought it looked good. When finished, the new legs looked great, and the exposed steel was painted red. When I put them on the first time, I immediately noticed a huge weight difference compared to the previous pair. I was surprised how much weight was decreased by leaving out the extra outer layers. Not only did the legs weigh less, but so did the shoes. Because I was altogether impressed by how lightweight they were, it gave me new motivation to work with them more. It was actually Vicki's suggestion that I surprise everyone at camp by putting my prosthetics on during the dance. I didn't exactly like the idea of putting on a show and all those eyes being on me, but I did it anyway. When the night of the dance arrived, Joey helped me get them on, and with further help, I stood up at the dance for everyone to see. I got a lot of smiles and wide-eyed stares of amazement and shock like, "Wow, he's standing!" along with plenty of words of encouragement. I stood for a few minutes until I sat back down in my chair. Unfortunately, fate sometimes has cruel humor and a way of changing direction. Later that evening, one of the CITs did a handstand and ended up falling backward, hitting my leg. It could've happened to anyone, and I didn't blame him at all. At the end of the dance that year, we began an annual tradition by playing R. Kelly's hit "I believe I Can Fly." Camp is the one place where all our worries melt away and where we learn we have unlimited potential with the support of those who love and care. The message of the song is that we can do it because we believe in ourselves and each other. Ever since that first time it was played in '97, camp is never complete or over without playing it. As for my leg, it felt somewhat okay until bed, and then the pain just skyrocketed. I had my wheelchair next to my bunk, and I tried to elevate it as best I could. The pain was intense for a while, and I don't remember if I managed to get some Tylenol or not, but eventually, the pain subsided enough so I could get some sleep. Like I said, I don't blame him for it. Accidents happen, and at the time, I was worried that it might mean I was due for another amputation revision surgery on my legs. I did not look forward to any surgery, but I knew that more were inevitable, and another on my legs was quite likely to come. It was a great week that year at camp. It was always a great week, but being a CIT was a new, refreshing, and different way to experience and enjoy camp. And of course, going home was still just as difficult. Boarding the buses and departing seemed to drag on forever as we said our good-byes until yet another year; so many tears were falling from so many people as the buses drove off, and a very stressful although *fun* week was over.

Usually, I stayed with Joey at least one day after camp was over before I went home, but he was exhausted and needed time to unwind. Although the next day my grandma came down to take Cassandra and me to the train show and railroad days in Galesburg. I hadn't gone since the mid '80s, and it renewed the interest in trains like I had when I was a kid. I got a few railcars, and I hoped to eventually get them running on a layout. My new room would be big enough, but planning and doing are often two different things. Summer continued, and progress on the new house continued to drag on endlessly. The longer Kyle and I were forced to share a room the more we butted heads—If I wanted to watch TV then he didn't or he tried taking control of my PlayStation, etc. Sharing a room didn't make my belongings his, nor did his wants overrule mine and vice versa. Also, during the summer, Vicki and Lee spent most of their off-work time helping at the new house. The other kids usually went with them, and Kyle and I normally stayed at home. In the morning, the nurses would come at various times for my morning shower. Everyone knows most teenagers enjoy their sleep, and Kyle and I were no exception. But the nurses coming in at various times for my care was starting to annoy and affect Vicki's schedule, and my preference of sleeping in as well as going to bed when I'm good and ready instead of whenever the nurse showed up that particular day. It wasn't anything personal against the home nurses, and I had friendships with them, but I valued my morning sleep and the right to decide when I was ready for bed at night. The home nursing schedule was just a remnant of being in the hospital, and doing away with it made home life more normal as well as increasing my freedom of choice and independence. So when we did end the home nursing services, Vicki and Peggy took over as my main caregivers every morning and evening. But on at least one occasion or two, I think I already had a shower, and I was back in bed but ready and waiting to get up. Unfortunately, I was unaware that nobody was home except Kyle and me. He was literally dead asleep, and despite my frustrated yelling for anyone in the house, he wouldn't move. When Vicki did get back home, Kyle was chewed out for ignoring me, but that's just how he was back then.

When midsummer arrived, London Mills had its annual summer carnival. But the town of about 450 people is so small I honestly didn't think much of it. I heard there was going to be a country singer performing, but that kind of music just didn't interest me much at all. But when I found out the guy performing was Tom Wopat and I realized who he was, I was both surprised and excited. Tom played Luke Duke on *The Dukes of Hazzard*, and I just couldn't believe he was coming to that little town. He was still an actor and singer, and yet he was gracious enough to take the time to play such a very small town with a population of less than five hundred people. I watched the show all the time when I was just a tiny kid, and the chance to meet somebody I saw as a hero from my earliest childhood years was like being that little kid all over again. A day or two before Tom Wopat's performance, Kyle and I went to the carnival, but there was a slightly younger boy making fun of Kyle pushing my wheelchair around, trying to start crap and just pestering us. The next night, we didn't want to go because we simply didn't want to deal with the drama and his mouth. We weren't scared in the least, but when somebody is harassing you, it makes it difficult to actually enjoy being at the carnival. We did end up going that night, and eventually after the local police were contacted, Kyle and the other boy were ordered to stay away from each other. On that night, Tom finally did perform, and even though they weren't my style, I actually enjoyed most of his songs. When he was done, he took extra time to sign autographs for everyone, and while I was in line, he personally delivered an autographed cassette tape to me, and I thanked him. I still waited in line so I could get an autographed picture of him with the famous orange 1969 Dodge Charger, General Lee. I was so excited to personally meet him, and the first thing out of my mouth, I said, "I watched the show all the time when I was little." *The Dukes of Hazzard* stands out more than any other show I watched back then. I liked *Scooby Doo* as one of my favorites at an early age, but even my favorite cartoons didn't seem to match up to how much I liked *The Dukes of Hazzard* or my memories of it. Those earliest memories are of me playing with a plastic General Lee or on the riding toy version of the orange car. As long as the show was on the air, it pretty much dominated my interest until it ended, and sadly, we all moved on to other shows and interests. But that show will always stand out in my memory as my first favorite, so you can see why meeting Tom was an awesome experience. The older we get, it seems very few things bring back that magic and awe we felt during childhood, but I'll honestly never let that part of me fade.

The carnival and Tom Wopat was awesome, but the next few days afterwards, I was increasingly worried about my cat Max. He was allowed to roam outdoors and was sometimes gone a day or two, but the days since I had seen him last were adding up. The longer it went, the more certain I felt that he wasn't coming back. I thought to myself, *Well, he was with me for four years, longer than any previous pet, and I'll miss him.* I wondered if he got hit by a car, maybe a coyote got him, or perhaps a neighbor took a shot at him with a pellet gun. Two weeks had passed, and I was unaware that Vicki put up a missing cat photo at the post office in town. It wasn't much longer when Vicki got a tip from somebody in town who may have found him but didn't actually have him at that moment. A lady in town who put food out for her own cats noticed that the food was running out quickly and eventually discovered Max. Somehow he managed to walk about a mile, cross a lone bridge into town, but couldn't find his way back. We could hear the music and see the lights all the way out at our place, so we just assumed Max's curiosity got the best of him when he decided to search out where the noise was coming from. I went from being certain that he was gone for good and then suddenly thankful and relieved when he was found. I felt like one of those lucky pet owners whose pet had been missing for a year or more and travelled cross-country to reunite. It had been a little over two weeks, but after believing he was gone for good, it seemed like forever. I was thankful to the person who found him, and even Max seemed glad to be home with his own bowl of cat food, a roof over his head, and a warm bed at night, my bed.

By late summer, I was once again in the final steps of acquiring a new power wheelchair. On average, Medicare will cover the cost of a new wheelchair about every five years or so. My wheelchair was almost seven years old already, and it was clearly showing its age. Over the years, it had been out of commission because of flat tires, broken drive belts, or water getting into the electronics. It was getting so bad that every now and then the controller would stick and the chair would start spinning until it was shut off. Whenever that happened, anything or anyone unfortunate enough to be in the spin zone was violently knocked or pushed out of the way, and quite often, my legs ended up taking a very painful hit or two. So clearly, the need for a new chair was becoming greater as time went on. Not only did I need the chair for mobility, but those involved with my medical needs and well-being all wanted a wheelchair better fitted for my scoliosis. At that point in time, I had no physical effects from the scoliosis other than no longer being able to rest my head on my knees, and when laid down on flatter surfaces, it was slowly becoming slightly harder for me to roll onto my right side. And though I wasn't yet feeling any physical effects, I was starting to see the curvature in my spine when I saw my reflection in the bathroom mirror. It was on the wall in the bathroom facing the tub, and every shower, I had a reminder of my scoliosis *and* my appearance. The scoliosis was becoming more noticeable visually, and I hated that constant reminder of it when I saw my own reflection in the mirror. I'm not ashamed of my appearance or my scars, but I'm certainly conflicted sometimes because I may be proud of my scars and being a burn survivor, but I know I'm not the only one of "us" who often thinks back to how we looked before being burned.

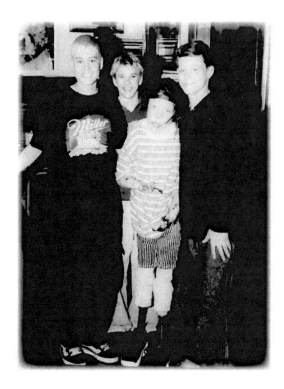

Chapter 32

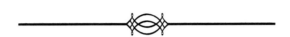

Before I knew it, the final weeks of August had arrived, summer was over, and my senior year in high school had finally begun. Taken from a song called "Lessons" by dBPony:

These lessons are surely my demise

Can't you see the boredom in my eyes?

This isn't fun it's prolonged agony

Lasting for an eternity

Once again, I was back to the same lessons and old boring routine, but that year was supposed to be different. Though it seemed like those school years would last forever, senior year signified the end of a stage in life before moving on into adulthood and the responsibilities that come with it. But almost immediately, even before my first IEP of the year, Vicki and other advisors of ours were already wondering about my graduation. I was on track with enough credits to graduate, but the school was still trying to avoid certain legal obligations if I graduated. At first, I was dead set on graduating with no doubts at all, but as the year progressed, I increasingly got the feeling that it might not happen for one reason or another. In the meantime, at home, Vicki and I mailed an application to CCI (Canine Companions for Independence) for a service dog. We had discussed the idea in the past, and now that I was getting older, we decided it might be the proper time to look into it. I don't fully remember when we applied, but not much later, we received an invitation to the CCI's regional training facility in Delaware, Ohio. The invitation focused on an interview with CCI staff in person to further and more accurately assess my needs and requirements for a service dog. I answered their questions vice versa and was shown around the facility. It was cool to see the puppies in the back and made me excited to hopefully be lucky enough to have one as my own companion in the future. One of the final things I remember about the initial interview was that the waiting list for a service dog was typically half a year to two years. But after the interview, I was soon accepted and thus placed on the waiting list for a proper match. When a dog had been found that they felt might match my needs and personality, I would be contacted, and the next step would begin.

After I was added to the CCI waiting list, I was then eagerly anticipating four important things over the course of the year. The first to check off that list was the arrival of my new wheelchair. It was just a week or two, perhaps three, before my new chair arrived when Kyle and I took the old chair on one last adventure, fondly known as the *mudding trip.* And I still had mud caked on it the next day at school. Kyle and Vicki had mentioned it before, and I wanted to finally see it for myself, so we went over the hill behind the house toward a creek to see an abandoned railroad tress. The hill was actually pretty steep and, of course, muddy. We made it all the way to the creek at the bottom of the other side, and I thought it would be cool to camp back there or build a dam, but it would be a major pain to haul anything down there to build it with. Because of how steep it was. I honestly don't know how we even managed to get my wheelchair back up the hill and back to the other side. But by the time we did get back home, Kyle was covered in mud, my chair obviously covered in mud, and an important piece of my joystick was missing. It was a small ring which kept the joystick centered when not in use.

It was important obviously because, without it, steering is next to impossible and I couldn't let go without losing control. It also made turning the chair back on next to impossible because the joystick had to be centered and neutral before it would move. Somehow we managed to rig something to get me by until my new chair arrived. When it did arrive, I was excited to have something new, yet it also meant adapting to how it "fit" me, and that wasn't as easy as you might think and is a big part of why I prefer not to get new wheelchairs that often. Taking so long to adapt to a new wheelchair, wheelchair longevity, the long application process for a new chair, and cost are the three main reasons I don't get a wheelchair exactly every five years. It takes that long to get comfortable, and there are still plenty of miles and life left in a wheelchair that's five years old, which relates to cost. Just because I can get a wheelchair every five years doesn't mean I should or necessarily need to. If I'm fine with what I have, I'll keep using it until it starts becoming unreliable or unusable. So much of what I use costs too much to discard without getting all I can out of it. The new wheelchair had a few major differences and advantages over the old one. The first visual difference was that my old chair had the large-rear-tire style, like a manual wheelchair, and it utilized a belt drive to move. I preferred the large-tire look, but the small tire on the new chair had an enclosed gearbox, which meant no exposed belt drive, no more broken belts. The smallest thing would snap the belt, but the new chair's gear drive ended that problem. The new one also had a reclining function as well as shock absorbers on the back of the chair. My only complaint was the simple fact that all four tires were non-inflated hard inserts. That meant no more popped tires, but unfortunately, I also felt the tiniest bump, which made the ride less comfortable, and I did ask for inflated tires more than once, but my requests always fell on deaf ears, and I never did get any. But at least it had great speed and was even faster than the old one. The speed and torque was so good I could stop full speed on a rock and scrape it across the pavement. That was my mark; Caper was here.

I admit Kyle and I did get along sometimes, but conflict is inevitable, especially with him. Back then, you just never knew what could set him off, and I felt sorry for every new foster kid who came into our home and got on his bad side. But the same evening I returned home with Vicki after buying *Star Wars: Rebel Assault II* for my PlayStation was what I refer to as "the incident." It's in the past. What's done is done, and we all have moments when we are at our worst that we're not proud of. It's stuff like this that I'm not proud of and conflicted whether to write about, but it's the truth and part of my story nonetheless. These things I worry about pissing off those who were involved, but it's in the past, and we've all moved on. It began one early evening when Vicki and Lee had gone up to the other house, checking on something there. I wasn't playing my new game yet because Kyle was unaware I had bought it and I wanted the chance to play a bit before he took over like he typically did when I got a new game. We were in the kitchen, and I honestly don't remember what the argument was about, but he got next to me in my face, and neither of us would back down. It's kind of a guy thing, but I had taken enough crap in my past that I wasn't putting up with it, and I also wasn't afraid of the physical threat because I'd already been through hell and real pain. I didn't think he was dumb enough to actually injure me in any way other than a shoulder punch, and we both knew he'd be in serious trouble if he ever did dare do something physical to me. But the situation skyrocketed after Cassandra came over to back me up, which only pissed Kyle off further, and he then had a target he was willing to hit. So he lost what little self-control he had and started punching my sister until Mystic came in the room, and he began beating her as well. When Kyle switched his focus to Mystic, I told Cassandra to call 911. I know it was the adrenaline, but I wanted so bad to get out of that chair and beat his ass. It all went by so fast I don't remember who arrived first, Vicki or the police. But Kyle was arrested, and after all had calmed down, I realized what happened had the potential to get me removed from the foster home to another, and all night I worried about the possibilities as I regretted my actions. I could have backed down sooner, but the adrenaline and being in the moment sometimes pushes a person too far. When Vicki and I picked him up from the station, I said I was sorry and regretted what happened, but Kyle on the other hand was still too stubborn to admit that. I don't blame him, because he had spent the night in jail after all, and I'm sure his anger was still high from what transpired that evening. That is the worst memory I have of Kyle and me, but somehow despite our differences and his temper, we always eventually got over it after enough time had passed. For example, one of the funniest memories I have of Kyle and I from our mid-teens is when we were following Vicki in the mall, and as we were going by one of the major department stores, he jokingly grabbed a pair of boots and put them on the end of my legs. I looked stupid, and I was like, "Knock it off!" But before he could take them off, a polite and cute employee asked us if we needed help. Kyle was laughing, and he told her we were just joking around, and she saw I was an amputee, but she obviously didn't feel as awkward as we did because she just laughed, grabbed another pair, and said, "These might look better." Humor is important, folks. She ignored my obvious disability by humoring the situation and simply took it all in stride.

The second to be checked off my list of things I was most looking forward to was moving day. A year and a half after we put the Rapatee house up for sale, we were finally going to move into the new place. I was so ready to have my own room again. The only downside of moving day was the fact that it was the same weekend as my eighteenth birthday. I had wanted to be there for moving day as my stuff was being moved into the new room, but Vicki felt that things would go faster if I went to Joey's for the weekend. I was somewhat conflicted because I wanted to be there during the actual move, and I assumed I'd miss out on my birthday by spending the weekend with the Spences' and Joey. And to be honest, Vicki wanting me out of the way didn't help my self-esteem. I try to avoid thinking that way, but I couldn't help but think she had a point, because I had no way to help during moving and that I was just a burden. I was actually pleasantly surprised by the Spences' and everything we did during my stay that weekend. I assumed it wouldn't be much of a birthday like the one from the year before. But I was happy that they went out of their way to make me feel welcome and effectively get my mind off missing moving day. The first thing we did on my birthday was watch Joey's football game at the high school, and just like the game I watched Victor play on my tenth birthday, the home team won. Afterward, for lunch we went to Happy Joe's. I've always loved that place, and because it was my birthday, I wasn't surprised when that loud siren went off and the staff came to the table and sang "Happy Birthday." I never understood why Vicki didn't like that place. The only time she tried it was the buffet. Perhaps for her it wasn't as good as ordering a fresh pizza, but it's been a favorite place of mine since I was very little. I remember we went to Target for a little shopping then watched movies back at their place. So my birthday actually was much better than I assumed it would be, and going home to a new room in a new house was a birthday present itself.

When I got back to the new house after being gone for my birthday and moving day, my room was ready and waiting for me. Finally, the day had come to see what I had waited and looked forward to for the past year and half. I was no longer forced to share a small and somewhat drafty room with Kyle. I could once again enjoy the privacy and ownership of having my own space as I did before all the chaos of moving had begun. I could do what I wanted in my space and not worry about anyone disrespecting what was mine. Yes, the house was still Vicki and Lee's, and I had to follow those rules, but my room was mine, but there would still be occasional moments when I would be forced to remind certain younger individuals of that fact. My old room in Rapatee didn't have much space after my waterbed took up about three-fourth or so of the room. The room itself was neither small nor big, but the waterbed indeed took up a lot of space. My room in the new place on the other hand was huge. My waterbed still took up a lot of space, but there was easily enough room for one and maybe even two more of the same size. To put it in size perspective, even with the waterbed, I probably still had the same square footage my old room had empty. I had my full-size entertainment center along the opposite wall of my bed and a table for a few things, as well as an enclosed computer desk. It also had a walk-in closet with multiple shelves for storing my stuff as well as my clothes. The ease of access to my clothes and increased storage space was a huge advantage itself. But to make things easier in terms of my daily care, my room also had its own private attached bathroom. It was probably double the size of the old bathroom, and because it indeed was attached, I no longer had to be "paraded" in front of anyone else in the house when I took a shower every day. With the attached bathroom, everything was how it was in Rapatee before we moved, but the difference was the actual space. My bedroom was at least twice as big as the old one, and even with the waterbed, I still had plenty of open floor space, and as I mentioned before, I hoped to make use of the space with a train layout. Everything about the room was designed with me in mind. I had my own ceiling fan, so I could keep cool easier. The light switches were within my reach, and the door handles were of the lever style so I could use them myself. And last but not least were my new entertainment options. Living in the country and being in a wheelchair are both factors when boredom is concerned. There are only so many things I can actively do in my idle time to keep me occupied. So the room had surround sound outlets built into it, and I had my own satellite receiver. The satellite alone was a huge plus for me. Back in Rapatee, we didn't even have cable and never had a perfectly clear channel reception. At best, we had five to ten channels with the roof antenna, but now with our satellite and TV antenna, we had over two hundred, maybe even three hundred, channels and all were crisp and clear except during poor weather. But the satellite going out during storms was worth it if it meant more channels and a clear picture in the meantime. Switching from a roof-top antenna to satellite was like switching from horse and buggy to driving a car. So many clear channels available to me were light years ahead of what I had back in Rapatee or any previous home for that matter. And finally, moving in was such a huge change from the living conditions we endured while waiting for the house to be finished. A lot of work and care went into the first house in Rapatee, and you could see it. Improvements and additions were gradually added to make the place their own, which I had come to call my home, but sometimes the needs of a family outgrow a home. I had lived at the house in Rapatee for three and half years, and now I was starting over yet again in a brand-new, better, and bigger place. Most of the time we moved when I was young, it meant switching schools. Changing schools was always stressful and harmful to self-esteem. Thankfully, we were still in the same district, but school problems might have been easier if I had been forced to change schools. For weeks, I looked forward to the end of lessons of every school day when I could be back in my room. It was just me alone with my thoughts as I finished any homework, watched a little TV, or listened to some Bon Jovi in peace without somebody ruining my bliss by asking me to turn it down or off. Finally, it seemed like I was slowly returning to the daily rituals and lifestyle I enjoyed before the moving chaos began. Only now those things were improved and better than they were before. In other words, at that point in time, I was on a roller coaster high, and I was enjoying the view at the top while it lasted. For example, the first change I didn't enjoy was when I came home from school to find my waterbed gone. It had been replaced with a home-style patient bed with a powered air mattress. To be totally honest, I hated that bed in more ways than one. Simply put, the waterbed, despite its large size, was more comfortable than the air mattress, but supposedly, somebody had complained that a waterbed was probably a bad idea for my scoliosis. Looking back at my sleep patterns, after getting the new bed, I still disagree with that assumption. If I had kept the waterbed, my scoliosis might not have worsened so much or as quickly, but I won't dwell on *what ifs*; it's all in the past. And secondly, the dang thing was fragile. If somebody sat on it, like most visitors to my room did, it eventually popped an air tube. The blown tube meant an annoying incessant clicking all night long while trying to sleep as it tried to constantly refill the air tube. *Hiss, hiss, click, hiss, click, hiss, click, hiss, click*, all freaking night long until it could be replaced. The hiss was the air filling up and the clicking supposedly some internal piece opening and closing to allow air into the tube. Of further disappointment, I must mention that before we moved, I was promised a huge yard with more room to finally raise some more ducks. I had gone over all the plans in my mind, but as we grow up, we inevitably learn that things don't always go as planned. We had our new house, so naturally I assumed I'd eventually get some new ducks after we had settled in, and after bringing the subject up a few times, I realized it wasn't going to happen, and the promise of raising a few ducks was broken. I never appreciated being told one thing just to make me happy one moment only to be disappointed with a *lie* at a later time. If you're going to say no, just say it. Don't say, "I don't know," or maybe just because you are avoiding it. I'd rather be told the truth than given a false promise, lie, or avoided because of laziness to say anything. I had looked at catalogs for duck and chicken breeds, etc., and nobody said anything until much later. Delaying the truth only makes the disappointment and anger of a broken promise that much worse.

Shortly after I turned eighteen, Vicki helped me start the process of applying for my social security benefits. Surprisingly, I didn't qualify for disability benefits, so I ended up receiving benefits due to my dad's death prior to my birth. After I began getting my benefits, Vicki then helped me open up my first checking account. My account included a free debit card along with the normal checks. I thought the whole process was cool because it was another step towards adulthood, independence, and last but not least, the funds needed for leisure or other things. For my birthday, I had been trying to get some more trains to begin the process of building my layout and new hobby. But Vicki and Peggy, at the time, had been constantly steering me away from that by suggesting my new room needed a new TV, which I thought was pointless because a new TV was simply out of my budget. But I eventually ended up getting a twenty-seven-inch Philips Magnavox with Vicki's help putting it on a payment plan. I don't know how I managed to get by with the puny thirteen-inch TV I had before. So I was glad for their suggestion and helping me actually acquire it. Thanksgiving that year was completely different the previous years. Vicki's boss had developed an ongoing relationship with a lady named Cheryl from Ohio. Vicki had also become friends with her, and so we all ended up going to Ohio for Thanksgiving. It was a long drive, and we had to get up earlier than I preferred. We stopped at Cracker Barrel for breakfast in Champaign, Illinois, but I chose to stay in the van and sleep. I loved going out to eat, and Cracker Barrel was a rare treat, but the early morning meant my want/need for sleep outweighed any desire to have breakfast. I always loved turkey day, but along with the fact that we had to get up early, the other sucky part was that I didn't have my power chair. We had to take the old van simply because the van with my wheelchair lift didn't have enough seating. I didn't enjoy being immobile or spending the holiday away from home, but overall the trip wasn't bad, and Cheryl's cooking was at least as good as Vicki's.

At school, needless to say, the drama behind the scenes was still ongoing. Vicki and I had advisors, and other people acting on my behalf who were helping us deal with the school situation. At the time, so much was happening it was sometimes difficult to understand all the things that weren't being done by the school. In late November, Vicki and I went to a disabilities convention in Oak Brook, Illinois, much like the previous one I went to in Springfield. There was one particular seminar we attended that was for students with disabilities and included topics like overcoming obstacles to equal education, legal issues, and bullying. Near the end of the session, when the questions began, Vicki was the last person to say something. She mentioned a little bit about the bullying and ongoing issues with the school and asked for any suggestions and advice. Unfortunately, the answer and reply was rather rushed, and we still had more questions than answers. At this point, Vicki and I still didn't fully grasp the situation with my school, and I for one was still set and ready for my upcoming graduation in May. Even though I don't remember learning much from the convention, it was still a break from school and a nice getaway from the routine at home. While in Oak Brook, Vicki and I also did a little pre-Christmas shopping at Oak Brook Center just across the street from the hotel. Back then, we didn't have any fancy outdoor malls downstate, so it was much different than anywhere we usually shopped back home. Even though it was cold, the holiday decorations and being outdoors got me into a good mood for the upcoming holidays. But that wasn't the only fun part of our stay. It was also the first time I had the chance to hang out with Mara outside camp. I remember she mentioned prior at camp that she liked steak as I did, so I originally had hoped to go somewhere for dinner the night we met up. I don't remember exactly why, but the steak dinner was a no-go. I honestly didn't mind though, because living downstate away from the majority of my camp family meant limited time and opportunities to spend with them even just to talk.

So when I do have the chance to spend time with them, I'm always grateful no matter what the setting might be.

Unlike the previous year when we had no tree or decorations for Christmas, a little extra oomph was added for our first holiday season in the new house. We didn't go overboard with the outdoor lighting, but if it were up to me, the whole place would have been covered in lights, but the front porch, rear porch, and freshly planted pine tree in the front yard were all decorated with lights, so that was good enough for me. Vicki also took extra time to decorate the inside with lighted garland on the stairway banister and little festive things here and there. I even had a few things of my own to decorate my bedroom and show my own holiday spirit. It wasn't a lot, but I had my own lighted mini tree, ornaments, and Christmas stocking. But the highlight of the holiday was the return of our Christmas tree tradition we skipped the year before. Every year, I looked forward to the search for that one perfect tree at Grady's Christmas tree farm. When everyone was able to get along without bickering, it was a fun part of the holidays. The older everyone got, it seemed those fun and magical moments were fewer and far between. It was always cold and muddy as we got on the trailer, and the tractor pulling it took us out to look for a tree. But suffering in the cold was part of the fun because it made me anticipate the hot apple cider that waited until after a tree was found. Since we missed out the year before, Vicki said we could get a larger tree that year, and I was determined to make sure that's exactly what we did. The living room ceiling was twenty-eight feet tall, so the only thing limiting the actual size of the tree was getting it inside. The tree was so big Lee ended up being forced to trim the bottom off just so it could fit the tree stand, and even then, the top still had to be tied to the second floor balcony to keep it balanced and prevent it from falling over. If I remember right, I think the tree was at least thirteen to fourteen feet tall. We went to the Young Messiah Christmas Concert again that year, and somehow, it was even better than the year before. Out of all my memories at school, I look back at that one most fondly. Music is a powerful tool for boosting your spirits, and I thought it was just amazing that a rural school like Spoon River Valley could pull off such a well-done performance. If only the upper school administration staff had been as dedicated to my fair education as the musical director was to the music program, perhaps my entire high school experience would have been a positive one. For some reason, that year Vicki suggested that we open our gifts on Christmas Eve. I was past the age of begging for a present to open before Christmas arrived and actually preferred to wait until the next day like it's supposed to be done. But everyone else was going to open theirs anyway, so I was forced to either join in or be left out. The main thing I remember receiving was the N scale model train I had tried to get for my birthday. I also received my copy of *Jurassic Park: The Lost World*, and after all the gifts were unwrapped, we all watched it in my room. That was the only occasion we all gathered for a movie in my room. I don't know why we watched it in my room, but I think it was because we didn't have a TV with closed captioning in the living room yet. I preferred the comfort of my room anyway, and I look back at that night and remember it as a memory of how it should always be during the holidays, everyone getting along peacefully without conflict, just enjoying the present without worrying about the future, nice and content.

January 25, 1998, the Denver Broncos won the Super Bowl! As I mentioned previously, when I was young, I didn't really have a proper father figure at a young age that played any sports with me. That meant I had a lack of interest and basic understanding of games like football and baseball. But around age eighteen or so, I was beginning to gain interest in football, and my interest in NASCAR at the time was still new and increasing as well. It was a great game, because after three Super Bowl losses over the previous fifteen years John Elway had finally led the Broncos to Super Bowl victory. In the immediate days after that, I was searching for Bronco's Super Bowl swag to support my team. Just a few short weeks later, I was back down to Galveston for another surgery. The painful hit to my leg the previous summer at camp suggested to me that it might be time for another amputation revision. I had one prior amputation revision back in 1993 after I had entered foster care. But this time, I knew what to expect and was prepared for the pain. I was so thankful for the relief morphine brought. Without it, the pain was as if the wrapping on my legs was slowly getting tighter and the pain increased gradually until it became unbearable. When it got to be too much and the time limit was past, *beep*, I pressed the button allowing self-control of my morphine. It was my first surgery in four years and my last while I was still in high school, and at the time, it was the longest I had gone without having a surgery since being burned. Whenever I was in the hospital in Galveston, I often found myself wondering what my classmates and everyone else might be doing back home at any given moment. Darren might be having lunch, Jen might be in history class, or maybe somebody else was earning a free afternoon detention, courtesy of Mr. Tasker. Many students liked to give the guy a hard time and push the boundaries, thus earning a reprimand, but it was mostly harmless. And then my mind would shift back to myself as I realized what everyone else is doing in comparison to my daily life in the hospital was such a world apart. Many people just see scars and the fact that, at same point, I've obviously been hospitalized. There's way more to it than that. We face challenges for the rest of our lives, physically, mentally, and socially. Most people will never realize the various challenges and difficulties a burn survivor endures over time. At school, a student might be worried about how they look, act, or even their grades, but in the hospital, boredom, pain, and the constant longing for home and normal life dominated my thoughts. So many hidden challenges and difficulties nobody can see or imagine and that I live through every day have over time simply become part of my life routine. Something even as simple as a shower or bath in the hospital is a long and sometimes painful process and could require multiple nurses helping, while any other able-bodied person could simply step in a shower and be done with it, totally oblivious to how easy it is for them. Even relationships and friendships with other people don't come easy. But making friends and forming relationships can be hard for many survivors due to various reasons. For me, I find it difficult for multiple reasons. First and foremost, my hearing makes it difficult to socialize comfortably, so sometimes I seem like a loner. But I've always been somewhat shy and a natural introvert. I do like to be around people, but I'm not always comfortable speaking in a group. There are just so many things that present a challenge to me and other burn survivors that I can't even list them all. Even my caretakers face challenges, and unless you've helped a burn patient or helped to take care of somebody with special needs and/or disabilities, then many people don't understand just how difficult it can be. They often face their own set of burdens out of devotion to the one who requires their help and care.

On February 15, 1998, after nineteen years, Dale Earnhardt had finally won the Daytona 500 after coming close in previous races. It was an awesome and memorable race, and it was basically the Super Bowl post-game celebration all over again.

"Dale Earnhardt, what are your plans now that you have won the Daytona 500?"

"I'm going to Disney World"!

I don't remember the exact quote, but after the race, Dale mentioned John Elway and the Broncos and said something like, if they can do it after all these years, then so could he. Both events reaffirmed my faith and belief that good things indeed come to those who wait. The Broncos and Dale patiently persevered and eventually won in the end. Being a severe burn survivor requires patience for many things some folks wouldn't think twice about. So I tend to get annoyed when somebody calls me impatient. After all, I was eighteen and still waiting for behind the wheel training and among other things—whether or not all the confusion regarding my graduation would be ironed out.

As it always was during any hospital stay involving surgery, my time in Galveston lasted about a month. I was glad to be home, and surprisingly, I still had my hair. Usually, my head was shaved and the skin from my scalp was used as a donor site. But that time, the donor had come from a small spot on the back of my neck instead. This was perfectly fine with me, because it meant two less things to worry about, everyone staring and wondering about my bald head and growing my hair back to the length it was. Despite a few family and friends who had their own opinions about my long hair, I still loved it. I didn't grow my hair long just for looks or the fun of it. It also served a functional purpose and that was to cover the back and sides of my head where it couldn't grow. So gladly I still had my hair when I resumed school. The only real change was with my lower prosthetics. Obviously, because of the surgery on my legs, I wouldn't be able to wear them for a while until I had healed enough to tolerate them again. In a way, it was disappointing, because the previous summer had felt like such an achievement when I received my newer, lighter, and cooler-looking prosthetic legs, and so the surgery seemed like a setback. Sometimes there were setbacks when progress seemed to be gained, but that's just a fact of life for a burn survivor. That's how it had always been from the very start; sometimes I'd take one step forward only to take two steps back again. I would heal one pressure wound, and another opened up. It's a constant battle, and I savor the moments in time when my morning routine is faster because I have no wounds requiring care. Also of important mention, that spring was the arrival of yet another foster kid. His name was RJ, and like most of the kids that came and went, he had his quirks. I let him hang out in my room, and I admit I tended to torture him sometimes. Not in an evil way but rather an older brother teasing a younger one. To be honest, the kid was soft, squishy, and a magnet for punishment, but he also cried too easily for a boy his age. Yet he still managed to stick around long enough to be adopted until he moved out the following year. During which time, I got used to having him around. He could be annoying, and his talking back could get him into trouble sometimes. He was a pushover most of the time, but he still made himself heard when he wanted to be.

I don't remember exactly when, but the day I came home with my graduation brochure for ordering all the essentials to graduate was the beginning of a deeper realization that it probably wasn't going to happen. My grades and credits required for graduation were all fine, but the school still hadn't addressed the issues that they were supposed to and were hoping to be off the hook when I graduated. So when I brought home the brochure, Vicki didn't really say anything I didn't already know. And as the days ticked closer to the end of the semester and graduation day, we never ordered anything for my graduation. No invitations, no senior photos, no party, etc. Vicki was doing the right thing looking out for my future and well-being, and I knew that at the time, but it didn't make it any easier, and I couldn't help but feel disappointed and yet again left out. Sometime mid-spring, we went to see an attorney near St. Louis who specialized in advocacy for disabled students. During the interview, he asked a few questions about my background, the school, my needs, etc., but the interview came to a rather abrupt end when he asked one seemingly harmless question. The question was basically, "Do you want to graduate this year, or are you satisfied with your school?" It's not an exact quote, but I gave an honest answer, and my reply was I wanted to graduate this year even though I knew the school should do more. Immediately the interview was over, and he said I needed to be sure of what I wanted. To be honest, I'm still confused by so much of what was going on with anything and everything regarding the school, so you can be sure I was confused while it was actually happening at the time. Needless to say, I was the one who dealt with Vicki's anger because our trip had been for nothing. What could I say? I answered his question truthfully, but my full reply fell on deaf ears. Yes, I wanted to graduate *but* no I didn't want to forfeit what the school was required to provide by law. Late in the semester about a month or so before graduation, the thought occurred to me to contact Clare Howard from the *Peoria Journal Star*. I was over eighteen, so DCFS could no longer prevent me from talking to the press. The idea was to kind of update my life events since the initial interview with Clare years before, but most importantly, to share my story of why I wasn't going to graduate. It was going to be a wonderful article covering many angles, my daily life, school life, camp, and even my upcoming training at CCI (Canine Companions for Independence). I had just recently found out a month or so prior that they had already found a dog they felt would match up well with me, and my training was set to begin less than a month before high school graduation. But because I wasn't yet set to attend graduation, schoolwork wasn't really a priority at that point anyway.

Chapter 33

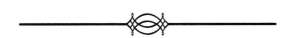

Just before Vicki and I headed to Ohio to begin my CCI training, I began a series of interviews with Clare Howard about multiple topics in my life, including high school and life in general. And then we arranged to meet in Ohio for CCI training and camp to cover both of those aspects as well. I was looking forward to the CCI training, and even though the experience was forever life-changing, it was also very exhausting. We stayed at a hotel about seven miles north, and class began early every day. If I remember correctly, we started around nine in the morning and usually finished at about three to four in the afternoon. It wasn't as bad as being in school, but nevertheless, it was still a lot of work. Training began with learning the basics of the dog commands and how their doggy mind works. Then we gradually began to ease into working with the dogs just to get acquainted. During the first week, the instructors watched us closely to observe us and see which dogs we seemed to work well and were most comfortable with. On Thursday, we were all asked to write down the names of our two favorite dogs. My first choice was Jaycee, and I honestly forget the name of my second choice. But the next day, as the leashes were handed over, I was given Jaycee. I was so excited to be paired with my first choice, because I knew we would make a great team, and so did my instructors.

The day we were paired with our dogs was also the first day we were allowed to take them to our hotel at the end of the day. I spent that first evening just chilling on the hotel bed, watching TV, but mostly bonding with Jaycee. Somehow, I was able to figure out how to get her to bark, and I spent a few hours that evening training her to speak. And amazingly, the hotel never did complain about her barking that night. The next morning in class, my instructors were stunned when I demonstrated to them that I had taught Jaycee to speak after only one night together. Even though they had tried to get her to speak, they never had the success like I did. As I mentioned earlier, the days were long, and Vicki and I had almost zero time apart during our two weeks of training, and inevitably, this led to a clash of personalities. One particular afternoon training session in the kennel area, we were asked to give the dogs a command, but apparently, I didn't react fast enough, and Vicki must have read a look on my face that wasn't there and dragged me outside, lectured me about my attitude, and threatened to go home. I honestly thought she was overreacting to something I didn't do, but I shrugged it off and moved on. The only other hiccup during our time training was also one of the most embarrassing. During our class sessions, we were told accidents in public would sometimes happen. The dogs were being tested in situations with us, and it was new for dog and person. I shrugged it off and never thought it would happen to us. Lo and behold, I was wrong. Our first trip to the mall during our class training trip, Jaycee proved we weren't invulnerable to statistics, to put it mildly. Thankfully, Vicki was there to help me out. And luckily, an accident when I was alone with Jaycee never happened during our time together. That truly would have been embarrassing, but I still would have been obligated to ask somebody for help. Leaving it there would be bad public relations for service dogs in general, but asking a random stranger to pick up her gift would have been just as awkward and embarrassing, as if I had done the dirty deed myself.

That same day at the mall outing, we visited one last shop. It was a gift style shop similar to Hallmark with ornaments, cards, ceramic statues, etc. As we were browsing, Jaycee suddenly froze in place as she stared at something. I then quickly noticed she had locked eyes with a life-size statue of a Labrador retriever. She was unsure of this strange stiff dog and wouldn't budge. Vicki then approached it and knocked it on the head. This eased her tension, and she slowly began to ease up to it. She carefully checked it out by sniffing and inspecting it the way dogs do until she was satisfied it wasn't a threat. That will always be one of my favorite early memories of Jaycee during our training. It was so funny when I noticed her reaction to that statue. Not all that different from a toddler being scared of Santa or the Easter Bunny. On the other hand, one of the biggest challenges during our training was our day trip to the Columbus Zoo. Not only was it a bit hot for me that day, but Jaycee apparently was making it known that she loved small animals. Out of her class, she probably had the most trouble paying attention when around small animals and particularly waterfowl, which put a lot of stress on my leash arm. Her trainers told me they never had a problem with her, so perhaps she assumed she could be a part-time hunting dog. Luckily for her, when we returned home, we had a friend's property with a secluded pond where she could run and swim for a few hours to run off extra energy sometimes. She really loved water, and that's an understatement. If we were sitting somewhere long enough where she had a view of a lake—for example, at camp—she eventually grew antsy and whined and begged to be let loose. It was annoying and yet at the same time also funny just how much she loved the water. So she deserved to indulge when she had the chance.

During training, our class was introduced to a volunteer named Jim, whose wife had recently passed away. She was also a volunteer, and in her memory, Jim was going to donate the full training cost of $10,000. CCI is a nonprofit, and the dogs are free to those who need. All expenses are paid by donations from generous people. At the end of training, Jim chose to pay for Jaycee. During my time there, he saw in me my desire to live and love life despite what I've been through and, in turn, inspired him to appreciate his own life in a better light. Even though his wife was no longer with him, life goes on. Through his own generosity, her volunteer efforts would be remembered and appreciated. Even Jim's son who also attended the CCI graduation had generosity to share. Jim mentioned his son getting rid of an old outdated computer and asked if I might perhaps want it. His son overheard this and graciously offered to buy me a new computer instead. Generosity from people such as them whom I had only just met just goes to show that there is good in this world if you take the time to see it. And it's those good values, kindness, and positivity that I try my best to reciprocate any way I can. When people do something generous or kind for me, I feel it's my duty to share that with others and kind of pay it forward. Also of note, just before the ceremony, Vicki and I met Jaycee's puppy raisers Tom and Natalie. Jaycee's reaction upon seeing the pair who raised her was immediate. As soon as they entered the room, they both shouted, "Jaycee!" and the reaction was so precious. At that point, she wasn't on duty, and she was just a happy puppy again. Some people don't realize how deep a bond between a pet and its owner can be. But reunions like that need no words to show just how apparent it is and why those of us with pets see them as our own children. Talking with Tom and Natalie, I learned more about Jaycee's personality and what she was like as a puppy. One of the more interesting facts was that Jaycee would steal spoons and take them to her bed. So theoretically, her love of silverware influenced how comfortable she was with my prosthetics. My two weeks of training and finally taking home Jaycee was truly a life-changing experience. During CCI graduation, Shania Twain's "From This Moment On" played during a montage of photos from training and their puppy years. The words of the song perfectly matched up with the emotions of training and the future.

> From this moment life has begun
> From this moment you are the one
> Right beside you
> Is where I belong
> From this moment on
>
> From this moment I have been blessed
> I live only for your happiness
> And for your love I'd give my last breath
> From this moment on
>
> I give my hand to you with all my heart
> Can't wait to live my life with you, can't wait to start
> You and I will never be apart
> My dreams came true because of you
>
> From this moment as long as I live
> I will love you, I promise you this
> There is nothing I wouldn't give
> From this moment on

Those lyrics conveyed so much of what awaited in my years ahead with Jaycee. High school was about to end just as a new chapter in my life was about to begin. Jaycee literally and figuratively opened the door for me in so many ways. I can hardly begin to count how many ways my life changed by Jaycee being there with me. Obviously, she boosted my independence by helping me with tasks I couldn't do on my own, which also enabled me to spend the day at home alone for a few hours if need be. Not only did she increase my independence and confidence, but she also had a positive effect in social situations. Gradually, I noticed people of all ages were more willing to approach and talk to me. Instead of rude stares or ignoring me altogether, they would ask questions about Jaycee and me. One of my favorite memories was at Walmart when a little boy about three to four years old ran directly in front of me as I was quickly heading toward the exit. I stopped quickly and locked eyes with the boy's mom as a way of saying, "Don't worry, he scared me too, but I saw him." It was funny because the boy just ran directly for Jaycee as if I was totally invisible, and as if she had been in Walmart alone. Many elements were starting to fall into place in terms of my life after high school and my transition into adulthood and independence. Jaycee was the first "accomplishment" to be checked off that list. Without her, my independence would have been harder to reach, and my confidence to move on wouldn't have been so high. Things were quickly changing at that point in my life, and she was an essential and very positive catalyst in that change.

While we were in Ohio for training, Lee and Peggy did their best to keep things functioning at home. Unfortunately, my sister still had her issues and was being difficult like she normally was at the time. I didn't find out until much later that they had planned to come to my CCI graduation but couldn't make it because my sister refused to go. By then, I knew it was only a matter of time until she was eventually placed in a different home. I grew tired of her bad attitude and thought just maybe she might be happier and better off somewhere else. When we returned home from training, school was already down to the final two weeks. But for seniors, we only had a week of classes left. I did my best to catch up during the final days and hours doing extra work here and there, but it was pretty pointless, to be honest. When my final day arrived, I was basically given a free pass from any incomplete work and sent home early on the bus alone because I was the only senior who needed a ride. Vicki wasn't home, so I told the driver she could drop me off just down the road where she worked. At first, she was unaware, and I don't recall how I got her attention to come out, but she was surprised to see me waiting for her. I explained the situation, and despite all that, she still thought I should be at school finishing up on anything I had left. This is where it got awkward for me, and I started to get annoyed with everyone involved. I felt the school wanted one less student to transport, be responsible for, etc. And Vicki most likely was just too busy and not ready for summer to start. She had nobody available to help me out alone, so school would suffice until it was over. That's my theory at least, but the juggling back and forth pissed me off when all I wanted to do was stay home and enjoy my newfound independence with Jaycee. When I was at school, there were no other seniors around, and I felt out of place like I shouldn't be there. Everywhere I went, I could read the look on the faces of faculty and students that said, "We don't have anything for you to do, so why are you still here?" I wanted to yell out it wasn't my choice to be there. To put it bluntly, I still have nightmares of being sent to school even though it is logically pointless. It's hard to explain, but I think it has something to do with my subconscious believing that part of me will never be smart enough because of all the drama surrounding my education during the final years in high school. Most of the time, it involves being sent to relearn basic math as far back as second and third grade, even kindergarten. What's weird is some of them aren't really nightmares per se but more of a nostalgia thing. It'll be my present-age me revisiting my fourth- or third-grade class. I can go on and on describing in detail as over time these dreams have come to have a reality of their own. But in recent years, I've gotten better at fighting back in my dreams by explaining to authority how old I am (for example, as I write these words, I'm thirty-five), that I finished high school way back, etc. I explain I'm an adult now and that I couldn't be forced to do anything I didn't want to, especially something as embarrassing and juvenile as being sent back to elementary school because my now former elders and caretakers felt I lacked certain skills or couldn't accept that fact that despite my size and appearance I'm indeed all grown up. As a matter of fact, I also have similar dreams relating to health care I no longer require. Things like splints, facemasks, etc. that are supposed to be only temporary are forced upon for the simple fact that I'm a burn survivor. I try to explain that I only need a splint or face mask for six to nine months after a surgery, and I haven't needed them in years, but my logic falls on deaf ears.

After all the shuffling back and forth between school and home was over and I was officially out, I decided to spend the weekend with Joey. Paco was also graduating that weekend, and I very much wanted to go and support him. I was happy for him, and I couldn't help but wonder how it might have been if I had somehow attended Galesburg High School. Most likely, I would have been up on that stage with him, celebrating my own achievements. That day for me was bittersweet because even though I was able to see him graduate and his success, it was also the same day of my own graduation at Spoon River Valley High School. The entire time, I kept thinking I was missing my own graduation. Even though I wasn't present, my name was still announced in my absence, or so I heard. I should have been on that stage with my class, and I couldn't help but feel like a failure to my peers. Even though I had the credits and grades needed to pass, they couldn't possibly know that. So much of what I felt was because of what everyone thought of me. Perhaps they thought it was to be expected because I already faced so many obstacles with my disabilities that I just missed too much school, and another year was just a necessity because of that fact. But I flat out refused to let my burns and disability dictate my life, and my education was no exception. I truly wanted to be on that stage with the 1998 senior class, but due to circumstances beyond my control, it was in my best interest to forego attending my own graduation and thus began the legal issues with the school that would last most of the summer. I wondered what would happen next. Did I miss my own graduation for nothing? I certainly didn't want to go back another year, a big reason for that being I would be with the same class that gave me the most trouble during my time at Valley. Would I even be successful with the due process we filed against the school? If not then, I really would have been pissed and should have just gone on the stage with my class. I know it's rather cliché to say, but only time would decide what the future had planned for me. With the end of high school and Jaycee at my side, I was taking the first "steps" into adulthood, and I can honestly say that my life ahead looked brighter and better than before. I was just beginning a new phase in my life, and with it came a whole new set of challenges I was ready to embrace. My desire to succeed when some people said I couldn't gave me strength to keep going. The doctors gave me little chance of surviving my initial burns and said I probably wouldn't even make it to thirteen or even fifteen. I was now eighteen, still strong, and so thankful to God for giving me such a powerful survivor mentality, humor, camp friendships, and everything I've needed to continue on day after day. I won't let my burns and limitations dictate how I live my life, nor do I want pity or to be a burden. Even though sometimes I don't always see it, I have a purpose in life, which is always changing and evolving as the Lord sees fit. My appearance can fool people into assuming many things about who and even what I am. On the outside, I may appear to be damaged, scarred, and to some maybe even helpless, but on the inside, I'm a *soul uncharred*.

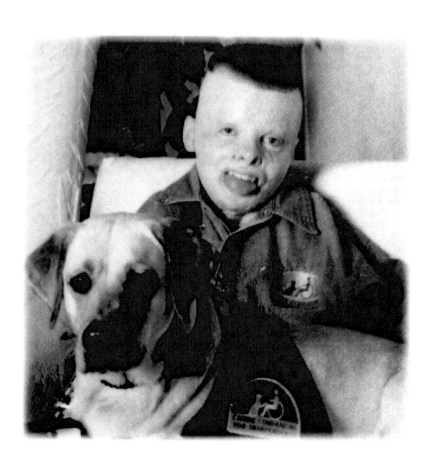

About the Author

Capernicus "Caper" Brown was severely burned in an explosion when he was just ten years old on April 19, 1990. From the very beginning, it was a miracle he survived. Doctors gave him almost no chance at surviving, and even if he did, they wondered what kind of life he could possibly have. Over the years, he's faced many difficulties and challenges that most people never face in life. He has also lost and missed out on things many people take for granted. Even during youth, he experienced difficulties of a different kind—the day-to-day struggle of growing up in a low-income family. He dealt with teasing for being poor before his burns, and after, he was teased and bullied because his appearance made different from everyone else. For years, countless friends and family have asked him, "How is your writing going? Have you started? Have you finished?" And now after all the years, he has finally got his experience typed out, and he's ready to share his story. He hopes to inspire others to see that life is always worth living. If you have an able body, that's all you need. You don't need to be thin, rich, pretty, smart, etc. to enjoy this life, but if you've got an able body, that's more than enough to enjoy life to the fullest. He also hopes that by sharing his painful life lesson, other people might learn from him and not repeat the same fateful mistake.

CPSIA information can be obtained
at www.ICGtesting.com
Printed in the USA
LVOW11s0348140317
527129LV00001B/64/P

9 781684 098750